ADD TEN
YEARS
TO YOUR
LIFE

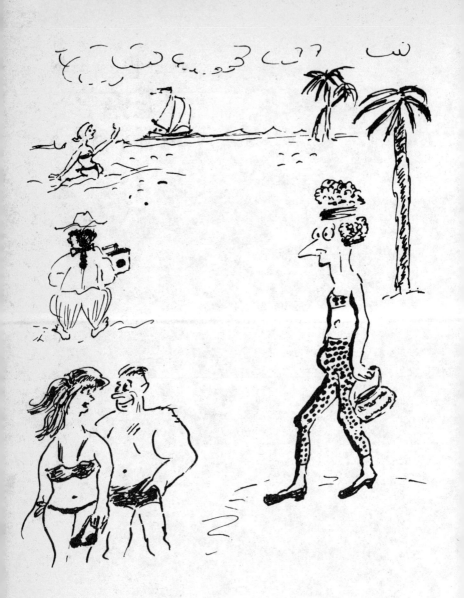

Stuart Trueman

ADD TEN
YEARS
TO YOUR
LIFE

M&S

McClelland & Stewart Inc.
The Canadian Publishers
481 University Avenue
Toronto, Ontario
M5G 2E9

Canadian Cataloguing in Publication Data
Trueman, Stuart, 1911–
    Add ten years to your life

ISBN 0-7710-8622-9
1. Canadian wit and humor (English).* I. Title.
PS8539.R85A74 1989   C813'.54   C89-094022-3
PR9199.3.T7A74 1989

Printed and bound in Canada

Books by Stuart Trueman

Cousin Elva, 1955;
reissued in 1977 in paperback

The Ordeal of John Gyles, 1966;
reissued in 1973 in paperback;
again reissued in 1984 (New Brunswick
Bicentennial Edition)

You're Only As Old As You Act, 1969;
Stephen Leacock Award for Humour

An Intimate History of New Brunswick, 1970;
reissued in 1972 in paperback

My Life As a Rose-Breasted Grosbeak, 1972

The Fascinating World of New Brunswick, 1973;
reissued in 1980 in paperback

Ghost, Pirates and Treasure Trove, 1975;
reissued in 1981 in paperback

The Wild Life I've Led, 1976

Tall Tales and True Tales from Down East, 1979

The Colour of New Brunswick, 1981

Don't Let Them Smell the Lobsters Cooking, 1982;
reissued in 1983 in paperback

Life's Odd Moments, 1986

Favorite Recipes from Old New Brunswick Kitchens, 1983;
Mildred Trueman's Heritage Cookbook, 1985

Contents

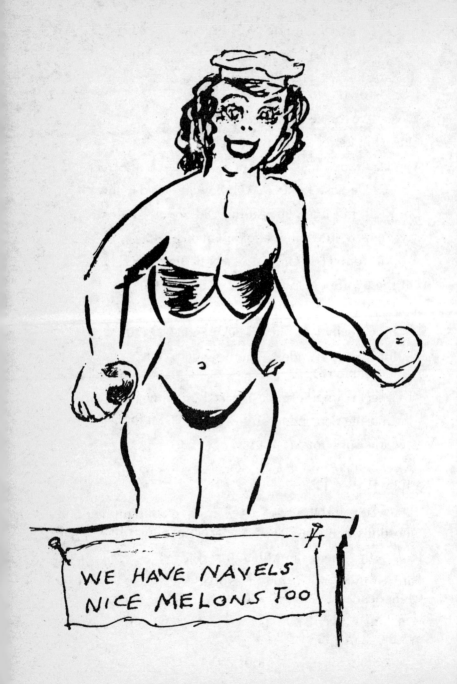

The Merry-making Widows of Florida

They are big, they are buxom, those hilarious widows over eighty years old telling off-colour stories just outside the louvred shutters of our condominium sun porch, where I am trying to write. Several are holding hands to keep others from capsizing to the lawn in paroxysms of laughter.

As any sensible person knows, ladies of that age should be sitting in rocking chairs on a veranda, tatting and speaking in querulous happy tones about their grand-children. They should be wearing lace caps on their heads, and velvet neck rings with cameo brooches in the middle.

But these high-spirited story-telling women refuse to abide by the rules. They wear modern bouffant hair-dos, and thin, flowered blouses over short shorts that apparently are their swimwear.

Nothing delights them more than chortling over the absent-mindedness of old men.

Says one, "An eighty-two-year-old man was shambling along the corridor of the senior citizens' home when a seventy-nine-year-old woman came out of her room next door.

" 'Hello there, Mabel.' He smiled. 'Say, can you guess how old I am?'

"She replied, 'Step into my room.' " He did and she shut the door.

" 'Now,' she said, 'drop your pants.'

"He did, and she said, 'Now your underpants.' They fell to the floor.

" 'Now,' she said, 'turn around and face me.'

"He did, and she studied him for a few minutes.

"Finally she said, 'Eighty-two.'

" 'That's amazing!' he exclaimed. 'How did you know just by looking at me I'm eighty-two?'

"She said, 'You told me yesterday.' "

My wife suggested to me, "If you find you can't concentrate listening to them, why don't you go to your desk in the front room where it's quiet?"

"I can't," I replied. "I'd miss all the jokes."

But soon they're traipsing off merrily towards the pool, planning an inexpensive lunch afterwards on the way up to Clearwater to see a play.

Next morning I encounter an eighty-nine-year-old neighbour who hails from Cape Breton, Nova Scotia. He still drives to Florida himself, with only an occasional dent in his car, and I only wish I felt as nimble as he does.

Disconsolately, because it's on my mind, I mention in our conversation I hate dirty jokes, especially the ones where you can see the end coming a mile off. And that is the only kind that old ladies at some parties seemed able to tell.

He grins. "I'll tell you a good one. You can use it yourself."

Lord! I think. Here's another one coming. And from such a respected old gentleman!

"There was this man who was very much given to violent temper tantrums and profanity. One day the clergyman came to call, and the man's wife served tea.

"The man said, 'It's pretty warm in this house. I think

I'll go up to the landing and open the window.'

"When he came down the stairs, suddenly three snow-balls flew through the open window and splattered on the far wall. The man jumped up furious to his feet – and just as quickly his wife jumped up and held her hand over his mouth!"

"Yes," I say, waiting for the kick line.

"Well," my friend says, smiling, "isn't that a good one?"

"Is that the end of it?"

"Yes!" He beams. "That's the joke. Don't you get it? It shows how quick a woman can be!"

Hopelessly I blurt, "Say – that's a corker! A wonderful joke! I can tell it anywhere."

"That's right!" he says, enthused. "Or you can write about it!"

Well, perhaps he's right, because that's what I've just done.

Rest Rooms Conspire Against Me

"Having a wonderful trip – wish you were here," rhapsodize the postcards I mail on the 1,800-mile drive home to New Brunswick from Florida.

It's only a friendly salutation. I don't mean it. Not unless the recipient happens to be someone I dislike. Even then I'd hate to see anybody go through the same frustrations.

Oddly, some of my friends always report an uneventful trip home. Nothing ever happens to them. On the other hand a Saint John couple I know stayed overnight at a large southern motel of a famous chain and in the morning found a car window broken and everything stolen.

Worried by this, I tried to set up a $4.95 ball-shaped battery-run alarm siren on top of the garment bags in the back of our station wagon. It looked great. We tested it. If the bags were disturbed, even slightly, the device tipped over and the siren wailed.

The only drawback was that every time we tried to slam the rear door shut, the thing fell over. The scream started. Other guests peered out their doorways to wonder why a reasonably well-dressed senior citizen was burglarizing a car in broad daylight, apparently too senile to realize he should wait till dark.

We decided it wasn't worth all those accusing stares.

But what really exasperates me on the long trip south is the filthy condition of the lavatories in many U.S. roadside restaurants and in most service stations.

The average so-called "rest room" has no light bulb, no soap, no hot water, no paper towels or electric dryer, just a brown-stained sink and toilet bowl and wet floors.

And this happens even in one with a banner outside: "Clean Washrooms." Which really means "Reasonably Clean When We Opened at 7:00 A.M. Not Inspected Since."

That is, unless they are large state "welcome centres" with a couple of clean-up men. In that case one will be sleeping on the grass, the other leaning against a post outside and sizing you up as you approach, wondering whether you might be a member of the state highway commission. To be on the safe side, he will mutter, "Pretty day, sir."

Many rest areas are well advertised for miles in advance – particularly in Massachusetts. But as we hasten towards them, they prove to be just a curved segment off the main highway, with no "facilities," as the officials call them.

Better, I think, to have at least a couple of time-honoured outhouses, in the old-fashioned New Brunswick and northern Maine style, than nothing but a few scraggly bushes with a high wire fence beyond.

You always see the same sights when you drive hopefully into a Massachusetts "rest area." Two girls are coming out of the bushes looking red-faced, joking unnaturally loud with each other. They weren't looking for blueberries. They just had to go.

And on a snowy wintry day, it's embarrassing to see

a parked car in a rest area with the driver silently standing on the far side, his back to you, and casting furtive looks over his shoulder. He's not just counting snowflakes. He's hoping you'll stop staring his way.

If I seem to have a grudge against rest rooms – if I suspect them of deliberately conspiring against me on a trip – it's probably because of experiences in the past.

They're always making a fool out of me.

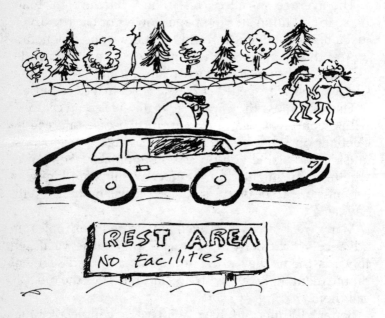

On several occasions I've walked innocently into a ladies' rest room. These errors weren't due entirely to absent-mindedness. The signs on rest-room doors these days look enough alike to fool the unwary.

I once gave a talk in Charlottetown, Prince Edward Island, before a large dinner gathering and then had to be rushed out, not because the listeners were fed up but to catch my plane for Saint John.

Unnerved, I dashed into the airport with only minutes to spare and hurried into the rest room with an apparently pants-clad sign. When I emerged, a station attendant said, "Were there any ladies in there?"

"No, why?"

"It's the ladies' lounge."

I wasn't so fortunate on the last drive up from Florida. Once, my thoughts far away, I walked into a washroom with a silhouette sign of someone in pants, and found a woman already sitting there.

"Oh, I'm sorry." I gulped. "Terribly sorry!"

She smiled. "That will be all right."

A strange experience, and a strange answer.

Another day I did a typical Benny Hill skit I had always thought too far-fetched to be believable. Looking for the washroom of a gas station, I paused and was about to turn back when I saw "MEN" on the doorway recessed by brickwork on both sides. I tried to turn the knob before I noticed "WO" before the "MEN." Luckily the knob wouldn't turn. The lady had locked herself in. She must have heard about me.

In Georgia, a gas station had only one washroom, marked: "MEN AND WOMEN."

I didn't try the door. I stood outside and asked loudly, "Anyone in here?"

"Yes," said a middle-pitched voice.

Uncomfortably I inquired, "Are you a man or a woman?"

No answer. I waited, and out came a pale young person with long hair, in blue jeans and a casual jacket. I still don't know.

To my amazement, when I went in I found no actual lock—just a wandering bolt held by three shingle nails, loose and pointing in all directions.

I reported this to the overalled man in charge. He looked at me, expressionless, handed me my change for the gas and said, "Y'all come back."

::

Why Don't They Ever Say Who They Are?

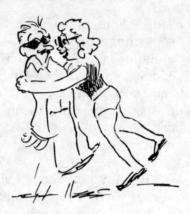

Even in this era of supposed ultra convenience, there are still serious problems waiting to be solved – some that our grandparents luckily didn't know.

For example, too many people today wear sunglasses.

A woman approaches me in a St. Petersburg supermarket and says, staring, "Do you remember me?"

"Oh, yes!" I reply glibly. "It's been a long time!" This is only partly a lie. It must have been a long time, because I can't place her in my mind.

But I wouldn't remember her anyway in that Lauren Bacall disguise. I wouldn't know my own wife in sunglasses.

"Do you remember the great fun we had at the Kingston hay-barn party?"

"Say, yes! Wasn't that a wonderful party to remember?" I'm still groping desperately for a clue.

"It sure was a zinger. And you finally married Amelda, didn't you?"

"Who's Amelda?"

"Don't kid me. Amelda Winters! The girl you went with four or five years."

Helplessly: "I don't think I know her."

"Aren't you Philip Snead?"

"No, I've never met him."

"And you didn't marry Amelda?"

"How could I marry her if I never met her?"

As she stomps off, still wearing her sunglasses, irate and feeling deliberately led astray, I take off my own sunglasses to watch her go. And I reflect that some women sure seem awfully silly to expect to be recognized when they're wearing dark glasses.

::

They Get Uplifted by Reading Church Notices

The plump Happiness Girls were back outside my sun-porch window, shrieking with laughter, but this time they were very aggravating. You see, on previous occasions the half-dozen over-eighty widows in shorts told jokes out loud, and shook so with mirth that two or three were holding one another's hands. I did see one fall flat, and it took everyone's efforts to raise her off the lawn.

But the trouble was now they weren't speaking out loud, just reading from sheets of paper, so I couldn't understand the jokes through our louvred shutters. It wasn't very thoughtful of them.

I persuaded my wife to go out the back door to clip and water the plants and find out what was happening. Dutifully she smiled at the group. "You're having a real laugh today. That must be great reading!"

"Oh," said an eighty-three-year-old, tears still dripping on her cheeks, "they're just a lot of church notices. We enjoy them so much. Here, take my sheet – we're on our way to the pool."

It struck me how very badly I had misjudged these good ladies. I thought they were always just out for a whoop-de-do good time; I'd forgotten that their early Sunday school training was still indelibly ingrained in them. Only a fool would have failed to notice that the St. Petersburg area is honeycombed with churches, and the huge parking areas are crammed with cars every Sunday.

My wife handed me the sheet when she came in.

"It's not just notices from one church," she said. "They've been collected from several different sources."

"That's lovely," I said. "They must be sort of Thoughts for Today."

"They sure are," she said.

Then I began to read the messages that had inspired our visitors with such ecclesiastical fervour:

> This afternoon there will be a meeting in the south and north ends of the church. Children will be baptized at both ends.

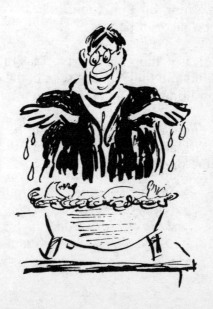

Tuesday at 4:00 P.M. there will be an ice-cream social. All ladies giving milk, please come early.

Wednesday, the Ladies Literary Society will meet. Mrs. Johnson will sing Put Me in My Little Bed accompanied by the pastor.

Thursday at 5:00 P.M. there will be a meeting of the Little Mothers' Club. All wishing to become Little Mothers will please meet the minister in his study.

This being Easter Sunday, we will ask Mrs. Johnson to come forward and lay an egg on the altar.

The service will close with "Little Drops of Water" – one of the ladies will start quietly and the rest of the congregation will join in.

On Sunday, a special collection will be taken to defray the expenses on the new carpet. All wishing to do something on the carpet, please come forward and get a piece of paper.

The ladies of the church have cast off clothing of every kind and they may be seen in the church basement on Friday afternoon.

This evening at 7:00 P.M. there will be a hymn sing in the park across from the church. Bring a blanket and come prepared to SIN.

Seventy-five Miles Without Seeing a Truck!

A re you a white-knuckle driver on those pellmell U.S. turnpikes?

Do you clench your jaws till your teeth ache?

Do you clutch the wheel in a commando death grip when you're crowded by racing traffic on both sides?

Especially when you see a sign ahead "Squeeze Right – Highway Construction" as if the foreman was confident that modern cars are made of rubber and can spring back into shape after a little fender-bending.

I can help you!

More than two million Canadians visit Florida every year – and most of the ones who travel by car come down from Ontario, because that's where Canada grows its biggest export crop of sun-seeking vacationists. They zoom down Route 75, after crossing from Windsor to Detroit.

An ideal fast trip – no tolls, no stoplights.

Other Ontarians and many Quebeckers follow a variety of zigzag routes southward.

From the more easterly sections of Ontario and Quebec – as well as all four Atlantic Provinces – a continuous stream of traffic drives down the eastern seaboard, mainly on interstate 95.

My wife and I follow a slightly varied path after crossing the little bridge from St. Stephen, New Brunswick, to Calais, Maine, and continuing via the short "Airline" route to Bangor, Maine.

The big difference comes when we leave the Massachusetts Turnpike and proceed a few miles along the New York Thruway. Then we turn left to drive down the winding Taconic State Parkway – a scenic wonderland bordered by little side-roads that lead to the upper-crust residences hidden away somewhere in the dense woods.

On an early November morning, after the first drop in temperature, the whole landscape sparkles like a frosted Christmas card. We see no trucks, just cars, on the seventy-five-mile run. Take-outs and gas stations are almost non-existent. At one, the old proprietor watches me from the window as I fill the tank. The quantity of gas doesn't register in his shop. So he picks up his trusty binoculars and studies the pump from afar.

He grunts with satisfaction, "Saves a few steps."

Coming off the Taconic, we find ourselves getting into New York and Pennsylvania Dutch country with its spotlessly tidy farms, tall silver silos like space shuttles ready to blast off, unusual barns with as many as sixteen tall, narrow shuttered windows irregularly spaced on the ends and sides, an occasional horse-drawn gig clip-clopping along.

No one ever forgets the overpowering scenery in the Shenandoah Valley, with the Blue Ridge Mountains towering to the sides as you travel the sweeping turns and hills of the deep-cut valley floor – a modern multi-lane highway with two or three lanes each way.

Crowds flock to the Shenandoah Valley's historic Civil War battle sites, where realistic mock clashes between South and North are staged every year.

Here's just an episode you may recall from seeing a TV

movie. Says the AAA guidebook:

"New Market (pop. 1,100). History was made at the Battle of New Market when, in May 1864, untried cadets from Virginia Military Institute in Lexington were instrumental in the defeat of a seasoned Union contingent. The boys' valor is commemorated in New Market Battlefield Park."

Perhaps Hollywood was back at its old habit of twisting history, but in the movie version I saw, the Union troops retreated rather than have to shoot at mere boys.

Eventually we begin to leave the mountain grandeur to travel past the pyramid-high hills of coal in the mining region, and finally the straight flat country south to Florida, where we get a sudden surprise at the first state "welcome centre": motorists with free glasses of orange or grapefruit juice in hand are strolling about in shirtsleeves. And I'm still wearing my topcoat!

We've escaped the paper-chase raceway through cities like Hartford, Connecticut. We've been spared the interminable traffic lights of little towns and villages. More important, we've avoided the road jams of Boston and New York and Richmond, Virginia, the need to take the Baltimore tunnel, and also the mad speedway bypassing Washington. And we've cut our road tolls in half, to about six dollars.

We've seen many strange sights, like the three tall, rustic crosses within view of the roadside – representing the crucifixion – that some religious zealot has erected all over the Carolina countryside as his life-work.

And big cultivated fields apparently covered with early snow. Really, the spectacle is caused by thousands of migrating snow geese foraging for kernels of corn and other grains left by the harvesting machines.

And those delightful Amish folk! Later I met three – two middle-aged men and a buxom woman – in a huge Seminole flea market, while we were waiting for the rain to stop. They were the cynosure of all eyes – because the

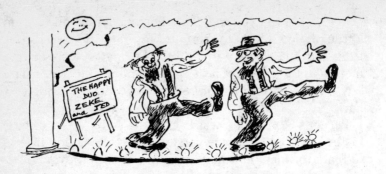

men looked exactly like Uncle Zeke and Cousin Jed from a 1920 burlesque show. They were clean-shaven except for goat-like beards that hung below their chins. One sported a straw hat with a wide, flat brim, the other an old black felt hat with a similar brim. They wore plain work shirts and baggy pants held up by heavy braces. The woman, under a sheer white voile bonnet, looked all the more portly because of her well-filled black blouse and full ankle-length skirts.

You wouldn't meet more amiable people anywhere, with ready smiles when you asked questions.

"How are things back in Pennsylvania?" I inquired.

"Indiana," the black felt hat responded. "We're here about a new Amish colony being planned in Florida."

"Is it still true you don't have modern electrical appliances? You know, like microwave ovens and vacuum cleaners? And you don't own automobiles?"

"Very true." He smiled.

"Then how did you get here?"

"We rented a car."

Gla
Sta
Geo

26 STUART TRUEMAN

as he stumbles out again. "You're g...
tation for scaring widows to death...
"I couldn't help it – I must...
"something else," he falters...
dark anyway." –...
"No. The front...
alike."
And now...
just for...
At...

...anada, I've
...out how my Florida
neighbour Georg......ngshaw, who hails from New
Brunswick, is surviving.

I don't mean under the muggy ninety-degree Fahrenheit heat, but under his wife Cressie's constant verbal
rasping.

George, you see, is in his eighties. He's getting a little
more absent-minded every year, as old men are entitled
to do.

But Cressie is under the impression that a barrage of
sharp words will straighten him up and he'll be alert
again.

For some reason, she only seems to make him more
rattled. Like when he returns home at night and gets out
of their parked car to enter their town house. He stumbles
into the doorway straight ahead, forgetting that his home
is three doors up the street.

"Eek!" shrieks Mrs. Altobelli, the pretty young widow
inside. I can hear the scream two doors away.

"You've got to stop that, you old idiot!" Cressie fumes

ing to get a repu-

ave been thinking about
'They're all the same in the

a shocked voice.

doors on our street. They all look exactly

— can you beat it! – she keeps giving him blazes
buying a few postage stamps.

least, that's how George puts it.

"Everybody needs stamps to mail letters," he reminded
me in a hurt voice when I dropped in.

Cressie intervened, "But not damnfool 'Love' stamps
he can't send to anybody but his granddaughter on Val-
entine's Day."

She held up a wad of unused "Love" stamps that the
U.S. post office produces in five different designs, so I
could see what happens when you let a damn idiot loose
in the post office.

"He's still got thirty-four of these stamps left from last
year's issue – enough to last his granddaughter until she's
forty-one, so what can he use them for? He can't send
'Love' when he's writing to the Ottawa income tax people, or to the Florida department that refused to give him
a driving licence, or to my own dear mother, because he's
always grousing she's a busybody that he can't stand."

To soothe the troubled waters, I said, "He could use
them on his payments to the Florida power company and
the phone company. They have machines now that open
the envelopes and the machines don't care if he loves
them or not."

Cressie looked at me admiringly. "That's a great idea!
How did you ever find it out?"

"Oh, I just sort of made some inquiries."

But I wasn't prepared for the storm that broke two days
later.

Cressie called me in and waved four long strips of ten stamps each before my eyes.

"Lookit what the old idiot's bought now! And I only left him sitting in the car outside the post office two minutes while I went in next door to look at a shoe sale!"

They were all beautifully designed, illustrated and colourfully lithographed stamps of twenty-five-cent U.S. denomination, and each bore a nice distinctive message.

"Just see these!" she exclaimed. " 'Love You, Dad!' and 'Love You, Mother!' Lord – his mother and father have been dead thirty years. And this one – 'Happy Birthday!', showing a decorated cake. He can never remember anyone's birthday, and never sends a card anyway."

She went on, "This big sky-rocket bursting stamp says 'Congratulations!' We don't even know anyone to congratulate. Well, George's niece Alice is having a baby soon – but she isn't married and she's trying to keep it quiet."

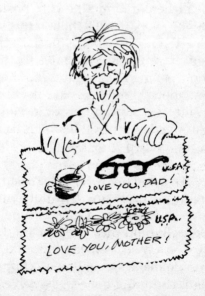

I suggested, "That's a nice stamp with the balloons that says 'Thank You.' Don't you ever thank someone?"

"No," she said. "No one sends us anything but bills."

"How about this 'Get Well'?"

She shook her head. "Anybody our age who's sick probably wouldn't last till the letter got there. The same goes for 'Keep In Touch!' I know what would happen. It wouldn't arrive until a week after the funeral."

By this time I realized the only way to prevent Cressie from blowing her top was to agree with her.

"You're right," I said. "They'd think George was studying to be a psychic."

On a sudden thought she commented pensively, "Why didn't they just do some nice ones with white lilies that say 'Deep Sympathy'? Now there's something we could use! We'd just put a little note inside, and wouldn't have to spend $1.50 on a card."

Long-suffering George interjected, "Well, I like them all, they're so pretty. I like to look at them. And besides, the postmaster here told me the U.S. postal department expects to make an extra $200 million this year from people who save them. That keeps postal expenses down, so they won't have to raise the rates too high."

"And who's paying the shot to keep the rates down?" Cressie demanded. "Brainless old idiots like you!"

"That's right, just nincompoops," I concurred. "Easy marks, push-overs, knuckleheads." Thank goodness George wasn't even paying attention. He was looking again at his lovely stamps.

It was just then that my wife, to extricate me, appeared in the doorway and said she had put some extra-nippy Canadian cheese cut up on a tray with new-type whole-wheat crackers. Would they drop in and try them?

Hurriedly I excused myself and said, "I'll pop in ahead – I want to make sure my news clippings and man-uscripts aren't cluttering the serving table."

Rushing into our apartment, I grabbed up my own

twelve long strips of the new embellished U.S. stamps off the table, also my forty remaining "Love" stamps in five different designs, and shoved them into my desk drawer.

To my wife I called, "Please *remember*, don't get into any conversation about U.S. stamps, no matter what anyone says! I'll explain later."

At that moment Cressie and George trooped in amid gladsome cries of hello and welcome.

"I've just had a lovely chat with your hubby," Cressie gushed. "My, was it ever nice to talk with a sensible man!"

My wife shot me a quick glance and replied, "Yes, it would be."

Will They Ever Find a Cure for Shopoholics?

Heaven knows I've continually given good advice to people at home: "If you're visiting Florida for a while, don't rush out and buy anything the first day. That's folly. You'll probably find it at a bargain price next day at another store."

I don't know how many people have taken this helpful counsel to heart.

Unhappily, I haven't.

I'm a confirmed shopoholic. I'm just fascinated by the glittering store displays.

We'd no sooner arrived from Canada than a letter came addressed to me personally. A big department store, newly redesigned and enlarged, was having a great "Pre-Thanksgiving Christmas Sale" next day. And this official, who signed his name, hoped we'd be among the special guests carrying the letter to receive 15-per-cent discount on anything in the store on the special day – from 8:00 A.M. onward, instead of the normal 10:00 A.M.

I was enthusiastic. Who could turn down such a warm-hearted invitation, especially when we needed to buy an extension telephone to leave in our Florida apartment?

Here we were, still a week before U.S. Thanksgiving Day, the last Thursday in November, and wonderful Christmas buys were already appearing!

I didn't know how the manager got my name as a distinguished citizen, but I was ready to admit he must know what he was talking about.

We arrived at the store's vast parking lot next morning at 8:30 A.M. – and we were amazed to find it jammed full. Customers bearing packages were pouring out of the store.

Everybody in town, it seemed, was a distinguished citizen.

Inside, all was chaos. Long line-ups stood before every cash register. The staff seemed largely new and un-trained. Some clerks couldn't find out the price of any-thing and kept running to turn over boxed things to see.

I stood an hour and a half with the phone in my hand as the twelfth customer in one line. It never moved. An elderly couple at the head of the line had apparently decided to stay for the day. They were arguing with the male clerk, who seemed frantic.

The main reason for the complete congestion, I found out, was that the computer system had broken down. The clerks were struggling with hand calculators. Most couldn't work the strange things; they were used to com-puters. Some were sweating, trying to do pen-and-paper arithmetic. It was worse. They'd forgotten all about it since grade four.

Finally I buttonholed a floor-walker as he squeezed past.

"You can go to any check-out," he assured me. "They'll take your money."

That pepped me up. I left the line, amid good wishes from my smiling new friends, and trekked all the way to the distant shoe check-out.

Only two people were ahead of me.
I waited patiently until I got to the front.
The glum-faced clerk pointed to a sign:

This Cash Register Is
Computerized For Shoes Only.

How could it be, when the computers weren't working? But it would be futile to ask.

So I headed for an adjoining wing of the store, still carrying my $49.50 phone. At the jewellery counter I asked a blonde young clerk rushing past, "Can your counter take payment for this?"

"Yes," she said, and was gone.

So I became number ten in that line of ladies, and watched warily for intruders.

You see, I remembered the time in another store's checkout line that I was number seven. Among many very plump customers wearing skin-tight stretch pants with their behinds almost dragging on the floor, I spied one woman, beet-faced and perspiring. Concerned, I said, "Would you like to go ahead of me in line, madam?" I stepped back. Five women jumped in. I was pushed back to number twelve.

But this 15-per-cent-off sale in the other big store was a new education in the wiliness of people trying to get ahead.

Husbands, I noted, were cheerfully aloof (to all appearances) as they waited for their wives. But they always struck up a conversation with a passing department head, hoping to learn that he came from the same state, or was a fellow lodge member, or deep-sea fisherman, in which case they hoped he might come over to the wildly busy girl and say, "Would you look after this gentleman, please?"

The middle-aged ladies in the line had to resort to strategy more subtle. One unnaturally smiling customer sauntered slowly up the line, saw someone she knew, carried on an animated conversation with her, and before I knew it she was standing right beside her and then moved in ahead of her. If anyone stared at her, she just looked up soulfully to the ceiling as though wondering whether she'd be in time for her important medical appointment.

Another lady at the very end of the line had jet-black dyed hair, a craggy face, gimlet eyes darting everywhere, and a loud voice. Soon everybody knew she had a store of her own, and couldn't waste all this time. Then, with one of those artificial smiles when the eyes don't smile, she strolled up outside the line, idly looking at novelties for sale, and finally leaned on the glass counter and made noisy quips about what a hectic day this was.

Eventually the head clerk turned and took her payment, just to get rid of her.

I must say I wasn't any nuisance at all, myself, except for announcing to everyone that this mess was a disgrace and they'd picked too many clerks right off the street.

"I'm regular staff, " retorted the blonde clerk striving to operate her hand calculator. "And I'm working my butt off for you guys."

"It's always a scandal trying to shop here," I announced to one and all. I'd already been in line two and a half hours, and getting served had become a game, a challenge, to me.

When I reached the number-one spot at long last, the blonde clerk got busy figuring out $49.50 minus 15 per cent plus 6 per cent tax.

Mercifully I didn't know then that the same GE phone would be on sale downtown the next day for 33 per cent off.

Nor that the store I'd spent the morning in would soon be advertising "savings now up to 50 per cent throughout the departments."

"Here you are, sir." The blonde clerk smiled, handing me my change and receipt. "Be sure and come back and see us tomorrow."

"Oh, yes – that's very nice of you," I said.

"I won't be here," she replied.

Yes, They're Sure Great Bargains—But I'm Not Buying

They haven't given up the ghost after all: The funeral homes are alive and kicking.

For months while I was strolling around tanned, hale, and hearty this spring, I didn't hear from one hard-sell Florida funeral home or a Heavenly Peace Cremation Society.

I couldn't understand it.

In other years, when I was making several visits to doctors for check-ups, all funeral places seemed to be sending me glowing circulars with my own name gold-printed on them, or phoning me personally to suggest a free visit to their Shangri-La.

Did they have spotters in unmarked cars outside the doctors' offices? Was I followed back to my apartment? I never found out.

Lord knows, there are so many doddery senior citizens in Florida that the spectre of fate haunts even the happiest of get-togethers.

My wife and I drove up to the Clearwater Beach Hotel for dinner with a Long Island couple we'd known for years. As we passed Serenity Gardens, the husband commented offhandedly, "We each have an itch."

This startled me. It made me uneasy. I said over my shoulder, "How long have you had an itch?"

"Four years."

"I've had mine two years," said his wife sitting beside him.

I was relieved that at least they were both in the back seat. At the restaurant I would be able to get my wife aside and warn her, "Wash your hands after every time they pass you anything. Don't shake hands with them."

In a strained attempt to make conversation, I called back, "Where do you itch?"

"Not itch. Niche. We each have a niche."

Even "niche" perplexed me. Wasn't that what Old West bad men nicked on their gun each time they shot someone?

"We decided to save money by arranging ahead of time for side-by-side burial places," he went on.

The thought still bothered me. When we got home I said to my wife, "It all somehow seems ghoulish."

"Not at all," she said. "It's planning ahead, like anything else. Like, for instance, planning your vacation."

"Some vacation," I said. "I wouldn't be back."

After days of writing crouched over a desk by an open window, I was stricken overnight with a painfully stiff back. It was agony to try to get out of bed; I had to be helped. Then, after finally getting straightened up, I had to walk slowly to the bathroom leaning backwards with my stomach away out, like Tyne Daly in TV's *Cagney and Lacey*, who seemed to be expecting for about two years.

My wife, a nurse who keeps an eagle eye on me, said, "Probably your kidneys are gone."

But I began to recover after two weeks of floor exercises. "Lie on your back and raise your legs slowly up high, in turn," a back doctor advised me. "As a variation, clasp each knee in turn and slowly bring it up to touch your chin."

This worked well, except for some reason my knee always ended a foot and a half from my chin. I'm sure I must have a high chin and low knee. I even thought of growing a beard to get them closer.

I improved steadily, and in any case, no one had seen me, except perhaps when I walked outside to our mailbox to send letters.

But how quickly the funeral emporiums found out! Three circulars came in the mail within days. I learned I could be buried normally, with a carved granite monument above; or in a niche with just an engraved brass plate on top, but close to statues of healthy-looking chubby cherubs; or cremated, with the ashes to be scattered at sea or on one's own favourite old place, like a hilltop. (One woman visitor grumbled, "If Sam had that choice, it would have to be the Seminole Lighthouse liquor store.")

The newest idea came in the latest circular addressed to me personally. It was from Majestic Tranquil Haven Gardens, St. Petersburg. They were offering "Special Prices Now" – pre-construction discounts for "the beautiful, above-ground Hall of Remembrance mausoleum, the magnificent kind of burial place favoured by Kings and Emperors of old."

And there was even a special free gift – a personalized engraved metal U.S. social security card of "indestructible golden brass-a-lite," replete with a spread-winged American eagle and a U.S. flag on each side.

One of the many advantages cited for this card: It "creates a good impression when applying for a new job, credit, government benefits, etc.: saves embarrassment of showing a ragged and dirty Social Security Card."

The prospectus continued: "For allowing a counsellor to provide you and your family with pre-planning information about mausoleums and pre-construction discounts for the Hall of Remembrance, you will receive your engraved brass-a-lite Social Security Card at absolutely no cost."

Well, as I'm only a Canadian visitor, and also anxious
to head for the peace of home before the phone calls start
again, I'll have to take a rain-check on my golden brass-
a-lite opportunity.

Though unhappily I'll never know whether I might
have been lucky enough to rest right between King Darius
and the Emperor Constantine.

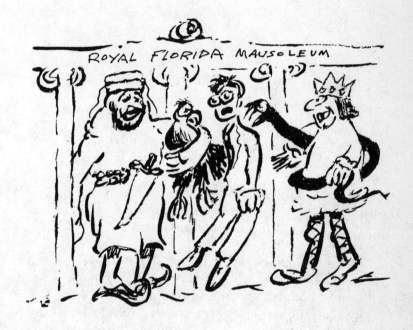

The Hazards of Asking Travellers: "Are You a Senior Citizen?"

Walking into a modern U.S. motel to register is a painful experience for me.

The pretty girl behind the counter says, "Just sign this card – and print your car licence number here."

That's the start of my embarrassments.

You see, I can never remember the number.

"I know it sounds like 'aids' but I'll have to go out and check it," I explain. The girl looks at me strangely.

I come back and say, attempting to smile, "AAD-320."

The thought suddenly strikes me: I should know my own licence number. Do you suppose she thinks it's a stolen car?

Then I ask, in growing befuddlement, "Do you have a discount for senior citizens? You know, for older people?"

"No," she replies, frowning at me as if wondering, How cheap can you get?

So at the next motel I don't even mention it.

"Do you happen to be a senior citizen?" the girl asks, writing.

"Yes."

"Then you should have told me. Now I have to make out a new slip, showing 10 per cent off."

Even when I do inquire, and they give me the discount, the day clerk next morning comments with a grin, "You could have got 10 per cent off your dinner last night and your breakfast, too, if you'd only said so at the time."

There's just no way of getting through it all comfortably.

If a clerk takes one glance at me and writes down "senior citizen," I'm offended. Do I look so decrepit there's no need to ask?

If, on the other hand, a clerk in a discount motel doesn't ask, and charges me full rate, I feel no better, though I realize I probably should be flattered at apparently looking under age. But I can't help suspecting it's the motel's policy to get away with a little extra whenever it can. I don't have enough nerve to make a fuss and show my senior citizen card.

Once, in West Virginia, when a doubtful clerk did ask, I scrambled to get the senior citizen card out of my wallet. I showed it to her. She said, "Okay." Not until I put it back did I realize I'd held out my Gold Club Member gasoline credit card.

This entire problem is one that affects not only today's senior citizens, but everybody of every age – because someday everyone will be up in that age bracket.

But desk clerks tell me they have the worst of the embarrassing job. As one said:

"People drive me up the wall. We're damned if we do and damned if we don't. Would you believe this? I said to a woman, 'Are you a senior citizen?' and she blew up completely. She said, 'Lord almighty, even my own mother isn't sixty-five until next month!' "

Out on a Limb

A man out strolling with his wife
    Puts little value on his life
If he makes the remark, of a girl in the park,
    "Say! Isn't that our Miss Fleggs?
But, no–those aren't her legs."

::

U.S. Education Crisis Is an Enormity, All Right

Television is often blamed for se-
ducing American kids away from
their school studies. Also needed, critics now agree, however, is less teaching by rote, more by stimulating classes
to tackle real-life problems.

As editorial editor Diane Steinle of the St. Petersburg
Times put it succinctly if not gently: "We're a nation of
nincompoops when it comes to mathematics." She added
that nearly half Pinellas County high-school students got
a D or an F in math last year.

She might have mentioned, too, that U.S. grammar
and spelling aren't very much better. The University of
Wisconsin handed out four thousand diplomas, but it
wasn't until six months later that a student noticed they
were issued by the University of "Wisconson."

And—horrors! As the votes surged in on that fateful
evening, newly elected President George Bush, the
"president of education," exulted on TV about the "enormity" of the Republican triumph.

According to the *Webster's Dictionary of the American*

Language on my desk in Florida, *enormity* is derived from several sources and it means: "(1) Great wickedness, as in 'the enormity of the crime'; (2) A monstrous or outrageous act; a very wicked crime."

When I told a prominent Florida Democrat what the President said, he smiled and remarked, "Well, there's a lot of truth in it."

Amazingly, a week later in his farewell speech, Ronald Reagan took pride in the "enormity" of the nation's development under his presidency.

"It just shows," commented my Democratic friend, "they must be both using the same speech writer."

Of course, you expect foreigners to make errors in English grammar occasionally. Like the boss of a Mexican dining place who told his patrons: "The manager can assure you he has personally passed all the water served in this restaurant."

However, another year of English is surely needed for the painter of the scrawled sign outside a condominium on a St. Petersburg beach:

NEW CONDOMS

FOR SALE

But not even a word was given about price, or whether you could get a better deal buying recycled ones.

These Dramatic Cures Aren't Helping Me One Bit

It's wonderful how many ailments you can cure in Florida in only six easy sessions.

The newspapers, TV, and radio are brimful of commercial pitches. You can stop smoking, stop drinking, stop being shy with the opposite sex, lose your fear of heights, lose weight, grow taller, sleep without snoring, become a macho man with bulging biceps, fly without fear, overcome impotence, banish claustrophobia, learn how to make your first million in your twenties (though you wonder why the lecturer didn't). To relieve aches and pains, two dozen acupuncturists with Oriental names are eager to stick barbs in your strategic places and enable you to scare your friends by going home looking like a porcupine.

Unfortunately I've found no advertised treatment here, hypnotic or otherwise, for my worst daily problem: feeling a draught and then sneezing uncontrollably.

I inherited this from an old-maid aunt who was very good at it. She'd even start sneezing when someone opened a window on the third floor above, or when she thought they did. When she screamed "*Achoo!*", our two cats scatted and wouldn't come back.

So in a restaurant, even with the windows shut, I have to sit away from the air-conditioning vents in the ceiling. Also away from big closed windows, which can transmit a cold chill to me in the heat of summer.

My wife, who loves fresh air, complains, "It's all in your mind. It's the way you were brought up. Why, the Florida temperature outside is eighty degrees Fahrenheit."

It *is* odd. Because on December days here I can sit out in the open wearing a swim-suit and reading the paper, without feeling any draughts, even when the mercury is dropping and passers-by say, "You'll catch your death! What a guy! You must be a snowbird from Canada."

::

Who's More Honest,
Americans or Us?

It was Georgia, the land of peaches and pecans, and we stopped for gas and a bag of pecans that first homeward day.

The gas island signs warned: "Pay Before You Pump."

I went into the convenience store and said to the woman in charge: "I don't know how much we need. How much should I pay?"

"Never mind," she said, "you don't need to."

This seemed to be a real compliment. Did I look so completely honest?

She explained, "It's only when I'm busy with customers in the store. I can't trust everybody who drives in for gas."

"You mean they come back and tell you the wrong amount?"

She looked at me sympathetically, as you would an innocent waif on the highway.

"They tell me nothing! They just take off."

I thought, "That's today's American youths for you. They rip people off and just laugh. Canadians wouldn't do that."

Then we went into the pecan store next door. The man in charge and his smiling wife gave us a warm greeting. Generously he cracked pecans and offered us samples to show how good they were.

He was middle-aged or over, with a smooth powder-white complexion that said he had never smoked or had a drink. His cheerful wife, more heavily set, had bangs.

The man wore a peaked cap; you expected to see "Jake's Auto Repairs" printed on it. Instead it said in red script "Jesus Saves," with a gold cross. Below this, "Lee Avenue Church."

Amazingly, he was cracking pecans between the thumb and forefinger of one hand. I can do two pecans together, and one finally cracks. I always thought that was pretty good.

"Here," he said, "try this paper-shell Desirable," handing half of it to me and eating the other half himself. "Aren't they tasty?"

"But isn't there a long shaped paper shell, too? Which do most people like?"

He sighed. "You may be thinking of the Mahan, over here. Try this one! It all depends on your taste. There are over 150 different kinds of pecans."

So we ended up buying a bag of each. I gave him a twenty-dollar American Express traveller's cheque.

The good man studied it closely, with his wife looking over his shoulder.

"U.S. funds," he finally told her.

"Yes, I can see."

When he gave me my change, I asked whether perhaps he didn't see many traveller's cheques.

"Oh, yes." He smiled. "Lots of them. But you see, we get a lot of Canadians here – we like the Canadians – and the other day a man bought $15 worth of pecans, gave me a traveller's cheque for $50, and I gave him $35 change.

"When I went to the bank, they pointed out it was a traveller's cheque payable in Canadian funds – and they gave me only $35 for it. So we lost $15 on the purchase."

His wife interceded helpfully, "He got $15 worth of pecans for nothing."

"We like the Canadians," reiterated the man. "It probably wasn't intended. It's possible the feller didn't realize he was handing out a Canadian cheque."

"Umph," I agreed, without feeling. What the devil was the stranger doing, anyway, travelling through the U.S. with Canadian travellers' cheques in his wallet?

"Well, thank you and come back again," the pecan man said, with his wife nodding smiling agreement. "Where are you folks from? Vermont?"

"No. Canada."

Their hospitable expressions didn't change, and I added, "We'll be back in the fall. I'll watch my traveller's cheques. But you'd better, too."

They even came out to the door to wave us a friendly goodbye.

Oh, for the Good Old Days When Lori Didn't Phone!

"Is this Mr. Trueman speaking?" asks a sweet young voice when I answer the phone.

"Yes," I say, puzzled.

"This is Lori!" She bubbles with eagerness. "Are you having a nice day?"

"Why, yes – yes, we are." I falter for words. I know in an instant I've met her somewhere, but I can't place when or where.

Probably she's the daughter of some Canadian friends of ours wintering here in Florida, and she's visiting them on Christmas vacation. No doubt I met her when she was just a toddler; everyone knows that if you turn your back for a moment on children today when you turn around again they're college seniors. Poor kid, she thinks I'll remember her.

To save her feelings, I remark, "Well, it's been a long time since I saw you."

"Oh," she says brightly. "In Wisconsin."

"No. I've never been in Wisconsin."

"That's funny. I've never been out of Wisconsin – not until three months ago when I came to St. Petersburg and took this job."

"What job?"

"I call numbers from the phone book to see if people want their carpets cleaned by the Holyoke Guarantee Company process."

"Oh." Relieved, my spirits start to pick up again. "Well, good luck with your job, Lori. We're not owners, only renters, so we don't need any carpets cleaned."

"It's done professionally. With steam cleaning and chemical shampoo, too. We have a special this week – only $24.95 for any living-room, dining-room, and hall!"

"That's great, but we don't need it."

"I forgot to mention it includes deep-soil extraction."

For a fleeting moment I think it might almost be worth $24.95 to tell her to send the crew, and get her off the phone. But then I remember my wife's undoubted reaction, and I wince. She'll begin in a moment anyway by staring me in the eye and saying: "Who is this Lori?"

In desperation I say, "Well, my bath-tub is running over, Lori. I have to go. So thank you for calling," and then lamely, "nice to hear from someone in Nebraska."

"Wisconsin."

"That's what I said."

"Think it over, and I'll call back tomorrow."

That's the bane of my life here. I can't break away from callers, women and men, who are so chummy and give only their first names and won't let me go.

How can I write back from Canada next spring to "Shirley" at the big department store and tell her the hand vacuum doesn't work again?

"What is your full name?" I had asked when I took it in for repairs this winter.

"Just ask for Shirley," she chirruped.

Do I address a letter to the store care of "Shirley, with

the dyed auburn hair and extra heavy turquoise eye shadow on the upper lid"?

The familiarity trend is growing every year here.

It's got so that I don't know anybody's last name – not just the phone callers, but also the bank tellers, the hospital nurses, the necktie sales clerks, the supermarket staffs.

Nor the young woman, Tana, who keeps phoning to see whether I'd be interested in pre-paying for a double burial lot in Sylvan Glades Memorial Haven.

She urges me to come and see the cemetery's glades myself. When I tell her I have a bandaged hand and can't drive, she happily offers to come and take me.

I can imagine the scene. Up to our town-house door, in this complex where so many old folks barely manage to survive, drives a hearse inscribed:

> SYLVAN GLADES
> MEMORIAL HAVEN
> When You Enter Into Rest,
> We'll Do The Rest.

Tana jumps out and says, "I came to pick up Mr. Trueman. Where is he?"

At every window, heads bow in sorrow.

Then, when I walk out the door and get into the front seat with her, old ladies faint dead away.

Just now another phone call has come. "I'm Barbara from Pest Control. Some of your neighbours have us come once a month," she says. "Would you like to have your pests exterminated?"

I certainly would.

Beginning with her.

How Ten Old Grumps Startled Me Awake

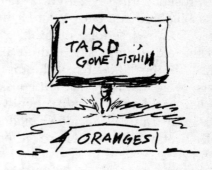

Thi he huge billboard said:

LARGO . . . 26 Miles
Home of 63,591 Nice People
and 10 Old Grumps

If anyone making the long trip from Canada to Florida was getting sleepily bleary behind the wheel, he perked right up. What did the sign mean? Who were the ten old grumps?

So you can see the wonderful therapeutic value of roadside signs in the U.S. South. They keep drivers awake, because vacationers either love them or hate them.

To those Clean Scenery Society zealots who would banish the endless billboards in Florida I would point out that here it's entirely different from home in Canada, where signs may blot out Nature's glorious views. On hundreds of miles of endless level Florida highways there's nothing more interesting to see than scraggly jack pine bordering the road.

But why, you may ask, would someone put up the Largo billboard anyway, and especially in next-door Pasco County instead of Pinellas County?

Very sensibly, City Commissioner James Miles answers: "Largo was tired of being ignored, downgraded, and confused with Key Largo farther south. And, besides, a billboard company offered the expensive space in Pasco County free for a month."

Will the old grumps sue? Not at all, says Miles. The statistics on the billboard, including the ten old fussbudgets, were just light-hearted guesses.

A friend told me he subsequently saw a billboard: "Welcome to Tampa, Suicide Capital of the U.S."

Well, that's Florida, where billboard craziness is contagious.

What I like especially are the little hand-scrawled roadside posters, like this one in northern Florida on a shutdown orange-selling booth:

Closed
I'm Tard

Nearby was a fruit stand with a painted sign:

We've Got Navels

My first reaction was: Haven't we all? That dealer should just walk the Redington public beach and see thousands of good ones. But it meant navel oranges, very scarce by May in St. Petersburg.

In rustic northern Florida we saw numerous men dozing in armchairs beside steaming table ovens: "Fresh Boiled Green Peanuts."

In a rural church driveway a man was excitedly holding a placard high over his head, facing traffic. I supposed it would say: "Repent, The End of the World Is Near." Instead:

Turkey Shoot 2 P.M.

Some posters you encounter are patty-cake innocent, like one outside a dinner spot:

This Is a Magic Sign:
Turn Your Car into a Restaurant

I'll always remember the characteristic graciousness of the highway speed warning as we entered Maryland:

Please Drive Gently

And this in the back window of a car just ahead of us in Florida. A printed warning sign, with a hand-scrawled message below it:

Baby on Board:
For Sale

North of Tampa is this billboard sponsored by a self-improvement institute:

If You Can't Read,
We Can Help You

But how could anyone read it if he couldn't read?

As we entered Florida from Alabama, we saw this billboard, painted by a worker who evidently could read but couldn't spell too well:

Welcme To Floirda

Everyone, in fact, likes to get into humour, intentional or otherwise. The dinner menu of the Olde World Cheese Shop in Seminole, referring to the Super Bowl game, said:

If the Washington Redskins Win,
Potato Skins Half-Price Monday Thru
Thursday. If the Denver Broncos Win,
Forget It.

On the side of a pest exterminator's truck in Seminole:

We Still Make Mouse Calls

In a Christmas tree lot at St. Petersburg:

> Genuine Northern Balsam Fir and Pine

I got a lift out of this. The trees probably came all the way from Ontario, Quebec, or the Maritime Provinces.

Pointing to the sign, I asked the proprietor, "How far north?"

"North Carolina," he replied.

Displayed outside a supermarket were beautiful Christmas trees. I heard a woman mentioning to her husband, "Canadian." So I examined the labels.

> "Authentic Reproductions of
> Canadian Firs and Pines."

And in tiny letters: "Made in South Korea."

Going through New York City, we passed a lonely old car parked on a side street. The sign in the window:

> Radio Stolen,
> Don't Bother

And some signs are a little on the mischievous side, to put it mildly. Like the lettering on a big transport men's wear van we passed:

> Haines Makes You Feel Good All Under

Or, at Starke in northern Florida outside an automobile radiator repair shop:

> The Best Place in Town To Take a Leak

But the first-prize winners, I think, were the ads for modern hotels in the small city of Intercourse, Pennsylvania, which appeared in travel publications.

Now, there's nothing wrong with intercourse. It's a respected old word. I well remember when I started as a daily newspaper reporter many years ago, prim spinster reporter Katie Broad finished many items such as parent-teacher meetings by typing: "On conclusion of the business session, the mothers and fathers enjoyed the remainder of the evening in social intercourse." They apparently always had a good attendance of fathers.

But some chain hotels in that Pennsylvania town seemed to exploit the name just slightly. Advertised one of them:

> Be sure and drop in to see us.
> We're right in the middle of Intercourse.

My first abashed thought: "I think I'll just wait, if you don't mind."

And some town stores do a land-office business in post-cards, which appeal especially to ageing grandparents to sent back to the family: "We Spent the Night in Intercourse."

That's how word usages change completely over the decades. A query about "making out" once meant how you did on your shopping trip or in your golf game. "Fruit" went into fruitcakes. "Making love" meant spooning, or, at the extreme, kissing.

I remember a magazine story I wrote in those days (I was slightly shaken when I read it again recently). It said: "She suddenly reappeared from her dressing room in a stunning abbreviated bathing suit. 'Wow!' he ejaculated."

Perhaps that's why the magazine never accepted another story from me.

My own real favourites, however, continue to be the unintended humorous signs you find here and there on the highways to Florida.

At a rest area where we stopped in the Carolinas, the green lawns outside the information centre were scrupulously landscaped. The highway authorities wanted to keep them that way.

One sign had an arrow pointing to the side of the building. It said:

> Rest Room

Beside it was another sign, in the path of the arrow:

> Use the Sidewalk

::

Florida's Climate Does Strange Things to People

I've noticed repeatedly: People who come into the balmy Florida sunshine begin to act peculiarly. The sun goes to their heads. There's no other way to account for their forgetfulness.

Look at Sam Gubbins, my neighbour from Manitoba who's in his early eighties.

Sam shuffles along the sidewalk towards the mailbox – and stops dead when he sees me standing outside my door. He stares at me, looking surprised, as if he'd never met me before.

I say helpfully, "Hello, Sam. You already got your mail about an hour ago."

But Sam, for all his memory lapses, is a quick thinker.

"Yes, but I got only a newspaper. I thought the postman might have come back with some letters." A moment later: "No, I guess he didn't."

And he shuffles back home, sometimes frontwards, sometimes sideways, sometimes backwards, depending on which way the wind is blowing.

Once he missed the mailbox completely and walked

over to the supermarket across the highway, thinking that's where he was going in the first place.

When we drop in at his home, and our wives are talking in the kitchen, Sam goes into the bathroom. Emerging, he looks perplexed.

"Did you see me go into the bathroom?"

"Yes," I reply.

"Did I take a pill?"

"I don't know. I didn't go into the bathroom with you."

This seems to annoy him. I'm not much of a friend.

Unfortunately, his wife, Flossie, has overheard. "That does it!" she proclaims. "From now on I count your pills and give you one a day." She adds grimly, "I'm sure you had four yesterday. You were up every hour all night, you old fool!"

After she goes back to the kitchen, Sam leans over and confides, "See what she's doing? She's trying to make me an old man before my time."

He reflects, "They say living in Florida adds ten years to your life. So I'm really about sixty-nine. I'm just a kid. I'm going to take up golf, like Jack Nicklaus."

And Sam let me in on a secret. The reason he may mistakenly seem forgetful at times, he explained, is not old age. It's just that he has too much on his mind. His wife has only the housework and the cleaning and the meals and the laundry to think about, whereas he has to worry about important things like the Soviet Union, and which pier will have the best fishing for sea trout and whiting the next day, and whether the Winnipeg Blue Bombers can ever do it again.

You can only sympathize with Sam and my other ageing friends. They will readily admit their wives are trying to reduce them to blithering old men – trying to do them in so the women can join the jollity of the sprightly, beautifully coiffed widows flitting everywhere in Florida.

The husbands are all wrong, of course. They shouldn't

blame their wives. The real culprit, I'm convinced, is the enervating sunshine.

Thank goodness I'm younger than Sam Gubbins, and physically strong enough to withstand the Florida climate. I have no memory problems myself; that is, none of any real consequence.

When we drove down to Redington Beach yesterday to stroll on the sand, I took along only sixty cents in change for the bridge tolls. I hid my wallet and credit card folder under two books on a living-room shelf, knowing burglars rarely stop to read books.

When we returned, my wife said, "Where did you put your money?"

After a moment I replied, "In a safe place." But I was beginning to feel puzzled.

"What safe place?" she insisted. "I hope not under your bed. That's the first place a burglar looks, you know."

"No," I said, frowning. "They're not under the bed."

As you see, I had all my marbles. I did such a good job I baffled the burglars and everyone else, including myself.

Anxiously I thought: Would I ever remember? Or would some workman twenty years from now, tearing down the walls to make room for yet another Florida high-rise, be surprised to find a cache of money stuffed in the air conditioner?

But—can you imagine?—just a few split seconds later my wife handed me my wallet and credit cards.

"How did you ever find them?"

"Because," she replied, "they were where you always hide them."

And my keys. Moments after I lay the ring of keys on the dining-room table these days, they disappear. As we can't leave the apartment without them, I grope frantically through my coats and pants hanging in the closet, realizing I just changed my clothes. No sign of keys.

Again, would you believe it?

My wife rummages around the same clothes, right after me – and plucks out the keys!

"You're getting just like Sam Gubbins," she says. "Old age is a state of mind, you know. You're even beginning to shuffle like him."

For emphasis, she reminds me I'm always looking around lately for my underwear – when I already have it on.

"It used to be," she adds resignedly, "you only looked for your glasses on your nose."

You can appreciate, then, what a relief it was to me when a Canadian neighbour's son, a schoolteacher in only his early forties, came to our door to tell us what a bargain he'd just got on a jacket in Clearwater during his Easter break.

"It was seventy-five dollars with pants," he exclaimed excitedly, "or one hundred without the pants."

We couldn't figure this one out before he rushed away to catch his plane home. And we haven't yet.

Next day I had a phone call from a relative I hadn't seen for twenty years, who was a teacher in Ontario. He and his wife wanted to drop in with their two children to say hello.

My immediate first thought was to hide the scissors lying beside my table lamp. The little tykes' grimy fingers might grab them and start cutting up the slip-covers.

Then the doorbell clanged, and I realized it was too late. They were already coming in.

And what a surprise! These "children" were a boy of sixteen, a girl of fourteen. They acted much more sedate than we did.

I'll never forget how happy that quick visit made me. Not only because they were congenial people, but also because when they were leaving, and the husband located the car keys in his pocket, his wife said: "You've got our condominium key, too, haven't you?"

He replied at last, abjectly, "I can't seem to find it."

"You've lost it again? After we got locked out yesterday? What on earth's the matter with you?"

It only proved my theory. The Florida sun had got to those two teachers, too—and in only one week!

Heady Brew from Vermont's Highlands

You can buy a little eight-and-a-half-ounce bottle of Ontario or Quebec maple syrup in a Florida supermarket for $3.23.

But in a long-established exotic food shop – where for about $3 you can purchase a can of Hobo Soup, or Buffalo Stew, or Pheasant with Dumplings, or Beans in Sauce with Wild Boar Meat – an eight-ounce can of maple syrup costs $6.95.

A Canadian visitor, studying the label, muttered aloud, "What a rip-off!"

"No," said a tourist standing beside him, "that's Vermont maple syrup. I live there and I know that our maple products are getting more expensive all the time. You see, we're losing maple trees right and left – nobody knows for sure whether it's caused by a blight or by acid rain."

Another customer shook his head sadly. "I used to tap my own maple trees on our Maine farm, and boil down the sap for the syrup. All for free."

He added, "I never imagined I'd live long enough to see maple syrup selling for more than fine imported Scotch."

Women Don't Understand about Bargain Hunting

It's a mistake to go shopping with your wife in Florida. Several New Brunswick husbands in this area heartily agree with me.

"They can't be made to realize," says my friend Ancil, "that our dollar isn't a dollar down here – that you have to add the exchange rate to the price tag. They buy before they think."

Adds his neighbour, Mr. Belson, "And also they have to pay 6 per cent sales tax here on clothing and shoes and books. But they keep exclaiming about the variety they get."

We all shake our heads in despair.

"Arlene made me take a thirty-mile round trip down into St. Petersburg just to save fifty cents on an advertised clutch purse," Ancil mourns. "I told her we used up three or four times that much in gas. She just replied, 'You said yourself that gas is cheap down here.' "

Poor Ancil. He knows when he's lost an argument.

I know how Ancil feels. I know, for instance, it's fatal to accompany my wife into a supermarket here. "Just for one minute – I only need a quart of milk," she says. To my dismay, I find her loading up a grocery cart with odd treats – "We may have Canadians dropping in this weekend."

Well, I think, at least she's spending her own money; she'll finally realize it when she falls short.

But amazingly after she asks me to hold the handle of the cart and start it through the check-out line while she hurries away to look for one more item, she disappears completely.

Before I know it, the check-out girl is beeping the groceries across the magic eye and telling me how much I owe her.

Not until I emerge with the bags piled high in the cart does my wife suddenly appear out of thin air, saying: "I wasn't able to find it after all."

Incidentally, one reason I can never locate her in the crowded store is that I'm convinced all the ladies of our generation in Florida go to the same hairdresser. They all look alike from the back.

Once when we were searching for an inexpensive wood frame to put a family picture in, neither of us could decide which was best. Finally, impatient, I carried one up towards the check-out, returned to the frame aisle, and found my wife still leaning over the display, holding up a frame.

Annoyed, I tapped her shoulder hard, and announced: "Are you satisfied?"

The woman wheeled around, her eyes piercing me. I'd never seen her before. She had chains hanging from her glasses, the kind that still scares former schoolboys.

"Sorry!" I said, and backed away. She was left to wonder whether I was sorry I accosted her, or sorry I paid for it.

More than once, as I slowly patrolled across the front of a supermarket, scanning each aisle for my missing wife, a cheery American oldster has said, "Whassa matter, fella? You look so sad!"

Unthinking, I reply, "I lost my wife."

Immediately he shakes my hand, frowning now, and presses my arm sympathetically.

A husband, I find, can't win even when he spots a real bargain himself.

"Wow – did you see this?" I say, looking up from the morning paper at my wife. "Scotty's is offering all sizes of frosted light bulbs for just five cents. The limit is three to a customer with coupon, and we have two coupons!"

"We've got extra bulbs now," she answers. "Six more bulbs? We're not staying here in Florida forever."

To my astonishment, she suddenly remembers all I've tried to teach her.

"You have to add the exchange," she says. "And don't forget, it's a round trip of eight miles. So it's no bargain, even if gas is cheaper."

Eventually, at my insistence, we go anyway. After all, I tell myself, I'll probably not be out more than a dollar.

Then it happens.

On the way back, my wife says, "Wait a minute! Isn't that a new shoe store just opening up?"

Reluctantly I accompany her into the parking lot. Sure enough, it's resplendent with opening-day bargains. And my wife eventually breezes out with a shoe bag.

"Was I ever lucky!" she exults. "They actually fitted my long, slim feet! I thought I'd better get two pairs while I was at it."

Now, I like to think I'm a very fair-minded husband. I refrain from calling my wife "Mrs. Marcos" in shoe stores any more, because for some reason she doesn't see it's a joke. Besides, I do remember how in past years I've hiked along with her to every footwear boutique in Toronto, Boston, and Washington in search of shoes that would exactly suit her hard-to-fit requirements, but to no avail.

But it bothered me to think that when I go out to buy a few light bulbs for five cents, I always end up by spending seventy dollars for something I'm told we urgently need.

It hurts a fellow's self-confidence. He becomes preoccupied, addle-minded. When later I went into a hardware store to buy a metal loop for the top of a lamp, known in the trade as a harp, I said to the saleslady:

"I'd like to have a harp."

"So would I," she said, eyeing me coldly. "But not until I'm ready to leave this earth. What do you really want?"

"He wants a loop that holds the shade for a table lamp," my wife puts in quickly.

That's why she insists on coming with me. She says I need somebody to explain things to people properly.

I well remember coming back to our apartment that day feeling pretty downcast. My wife, I thought, was still provoked at me for asking for a harp before my time.

To try to mollify her, I called the famed Kapok Tree restaurant to make a reservation for dinner.

The lilting voice of the receptionist, obviously English, said, "Yes, I have written your name down, love. Reservations for two."

"And what time would be suitable?" I asked. "Is six o'clock all right?"

"That would be a delightful time, love."

I hung up and said to my wife:

"Why couldn't you be that nice to me? Why, here in Florida they call me 'love' and they haven't even seen me!"

She replied:

"That's why."

It's Always Fair Weather When Forecasters Get Together

"**W**owee!" exclaimed the Tampa TV weatherman. "Eight o'clock in the morning, and another glorious spring day! Not a cloud in the sky!"

I glanced at the kitchen clock. He was right – exactly eight o'clock. And spring had arrived in March, so he was right on that count, too.

But not a cloud in the sky? This, I knew, was a head-on challenge to Fate. Even as he spoke, I could hear distant rumblings in the heavens.

The rain that followed was plain warning to all weather forecasters not to be so omniscient.

My fellow New Brunswicker Fred Quimby stormed in our front door, soaking wet. He was furious.

"That does it!" he cried. "Since January I've flipped a coin every morning, and I've been more accurate than the TV weatherman 60 per cent of the time."

Especially, he added, when that TV screen showed a smiling sun peeking out from behind clouds on every single day in the week ahead.

"That's always a sure sign," Quimby said, "to cancel your golf dates and beach picnics. Know what I think? They're all subsidized by the Florida Tourist Commission."

"Nonsense," I replied. "Forecasters have great professional pride. They wouldn't stoop to it. How can you suggest such a thing?"

"Because they're the only people in Florida who haven't gone to jail yet." He continued, "And they should, because they didn't give us more than two 'beach days' in succession all winter – except at Christmas, when I was up home anyway for a visit."

Sighing, he added, "Heaven knows I've tried my best to get dependable forecasts. I remember an old New Brunswick fisherman on Grand Manan who could foretell the day just by stepping outdoors. He could smell the weather, or feel it, he didn't know which, but he was always right. And some farmers would just wet one finger and hold it up in the early-morning air, and they'd know, too."

"There you are!" I said happily. You should give it a try!"

"I did," he answered sadly. "I wet my hand and kept it waving out the open kitchen window to get the full effect while I was having my coffee."

"And you got results?"

"Yes. Everyone going by on the sidewalk waved back. And car drivers grinned and tooted at me."

Quimby was in no mood, I could see, for me to remind him the Florida climate is fickle, that the sun can beam down in Tampa, thirty miles away, when we're having thunderbolts in Seminole. And, at the same moment the Gulf of Mexico shoreline, a mile on the other side of us, can be so chilly, clammy, and foggy you can't see your hand in front of your face.

He was determined not to be consoled.

I learned that, in a desperate effort to lift Fred out of the doldrums, old Amanda Hosbert had advised him:

"You always know it's going to rain when everyone you meet is grumpy. That's because ageing folks can feel the dampness in their bones. Especially Mrs. McKendrill – she's the fat one in her eighties with frizzled dyed blonde hair who loves to complain about her big toe. Just say to her any morning, friendly-like, 'Hello, Mrs. McKendrill – how is your big toe today?'"

Fred mulled it over thoughtfully. "Wouldn't 'Hello, doll' be even better?"

"Yes – great idea!"

But he seemed no happier next time I met him. He was limping.

"Why didn't you tell me?" he demanded. "There are at least ten women on our street who look exactly like that. The one I accosted was a Mrs. Polk, I believe, and she's a Tartar. There's nothing wrong with her big toe."

I had no alternative but to reveal my own infallible weather secret to Fred Quimby. He had forced it out of me.

"Keep your eye on Kathy, the little mail-carrier girl," I said. "If she's wearing those blue-grey long pants with a black stripe, it's sure to be chilly. If she's wearing blue-grey short shorts, it's going to be warm. If she's got the short sleeves of her blouse rolled up even higher, it's going to be extra warm."

"Yes," said Fred Quimby, "but what if it's going to rain?"

"Just peek in her little car while she's sorting. See if she has put her plastic raincoat in it."

"Gosh, thanks!"

Fred began rushing out whenever he saw the young post-woman's car coming. He studied her carefully all over, including her short sleeves to see whether they'd been rolled higher. He furtively peered into her packed car.

Sometimes he squatted, staring silently in a side window; then he'd squat on the other side. He never said anything to Kathy, because he didn't want to frighten her into hiding her raincoat, which would take away one of his clues.

That was, until two weeks ago. Then a fat, older female carrier with legs like telephone poles took Kathy's place. She always wore short pants.

Anxiously, Fred Quimby asked whether Kathy was on holidays or down with the flu.

"Dunno for sure," the plump one replied, "but she got a transfer. She complained, something about being bothered by a pain, but she didn't say where the pain was."

::

The Sweet Little Old Ladies Are After Me

Some people at home in Canada voiced reservations to me about spending the winter in Florida. They'd been reading about the frequent murders, about cocaine trafficking, about tourists pistol-whipped and robbed, about bribery and corruption in high public office.

"I guess you just never know when a stranger may accost you," said one concerned friend.

How right he was!

I'm accosted by strangers every time I go shopping here.

Many of them are cleverly disguised as sweet old ladies.

One sidled up to me in a big drug store. I was looking at a "coffee butler."

In a low voice she confided, "You can get them for two dollars less at the second shop down the mall."

"Oh, thank you."

"Uh-*huh*," she replied in a musical inflection, with a nod. That's what many people here say instead of the Canadian "You're welcome."

Was there a subtle sinister motive in her approach? I never found out.

But it seems to happen all the time.

I learned I was qualified to buy a huge white teddy bear, with colourful knitted toque and scarf and all, at a department store for only ten dollars after I'd spend thirty-five dollars on Christmas things there. I bought it as a gift to take home to New Brunswick.

Because my wife was still shopping, I had to carry the teddy bear in my arms around the big store.

Every elderly lady I met tilted her head, smiled happily, and nodded to me.

"I'll bet you'll keep it on your pillow every night," one remarked, perhaps with a trace of nostalgia.

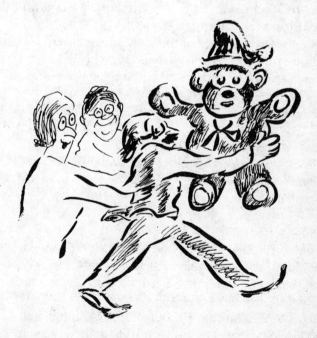

I found a box of four thermal plastic drinking glasses, patterned in different colourful designs, marked down from $8.99 to $4.97.

This was amazing – because I'd seen exactly the same glasses in a tourist boutique on Gulf Boulevard for sixteen dollars.

My wife and I knew the customer-service clerk, and when she saw us looking for a particular pattern we wanted, she came over.

"It's a real bargain," she said. "Better get a box while they're on sale."

Suddenly a middle-aged woman listening nearby put a cautionary hand on my arm.

"I wouldn't rush it," she said.

"But it's a bargain – it's on sale," expostulated our clerk friend.

The stranger shrugged. "I'd wait."

We decided to wait anyway, because we couldn't find the pattern we wanted.

When we walked out of the store, there was the stranger watching for us. Anyone who has read novels about criminal subterfuge would know instantly some Florida skulduggery was at work.

She said, "I didn't want to explain, because I could see you knew the saleswoman. I wanted to tell you that Walgreen's drug store had them on sale recently for $3.99. That's where I bought mine. Just watch their ads."

"That's good of you."

"Uh-*huh*."

We happened to be in Walgreen's the next week – and there was the design we wanted – at $4.99. So we bought it, realizing the stranger must have been mistaken.

But two weeks later, in a periodic Walgreen's sale, there they were – down to $3.99.

That's a peculiar thing about shoppers on this gulf "suncoast" of Florida. They all go out of their way to help and advise each other, almost as though in self-protection against the wild gyrations of store prices.

I was beginning to realize that perhaps, after all, on

this quiet side of Florida I didn't have to put my hand in my pants pocket and grasp my wallet tightly every time I was accosted.

"That's on the Miami side," a neighbour pointed out, "where the Colombians and other Hispanic drug dealers kill each other, and the blacks resent the newcomers' taking over their jobs, and the old established whites resent everybody."

It may be true. We live in a 159-apartment town house community where there apparently has never been an attempted break-in – possibly because a great ornamental sign facing the highway says: "Mission Oaks." This, we hope, convinces burglars driving by that we're all penniless retired priests.

We do often read in the newspapers here about brutal crimes; but when you stop to think that Florida in winter has twenty times the population of New Brunswick, the rate doesn't seem all that high. And sun-coast police have a remarkable record of tracking down crooks almost immediately, often from public tips.

My wife readily agrees with me. She never shared my suspicion anyway of strangers' overtures – which sometimes take such surprising turns.

In the vegetable-and-fruit department of the Publix supermarket across the highway from us, she was wondering what the price would be for one big purple onion (they were packaged in fours).

A passing woman shopper saw my wife opening the doorway of the grocery employee store-room and shouting, "Is anyone in there?"

"Just a minute," said the middle-aged stranger, taking over; "I've got a bar-room voice." She hollered in the doorway: "IS ANYONE IN THERE?"

No answer.

Then, as a last resort, my wife whistled – the same shrill piercing whistle she summons me with in a crowded store, because bellowing "Stuart!" would make everybody turn around.

From the other side of the department came the manager, running.

Fortunately there were no dogs in the store, or they'd have come galloping, too.

The other day we went to the K-Mart for their pre-Valentine flower sale – hundreds of pots of blooms.

Even as we stopped to glance at a front-of-the-store display, a woman shopper confided, "You'll find nicer ones in the garden shop through that far door."

For our apartment and its tiny outside garden we bought two geraniums in six-inch pots for $1.50 each, two pots of azaleas for $2.99, a pot of cyclamen at $1.97. There were all kinds of begonias at 77¢.

But I didn't expect the friendly reaction we got from other shoppers. They stopped continually to look in the shopping wagon and ask what we'd bought.

Advised a grandmotherly passer-by, "You'll need to give the geraniums some sun and a drink of water and fertilizer."

"Thank you," I said.

Another woman: "I wouldn't buy that forty-nine-cent pink plant. I had bad luck with them last year."

"Thanks very much."

A white-thatched retiree, wearing an Ohio peaked cap, grinned broadly when he saw me trundling my store cart. He exclaimed, "Why, Eliza Doolittle! How are your flower sales going today?"

I must confess I know little about flowers, except that tall-stemmed red roses cost eighty to one hundred dollars a dozen in New York, sixty to eighty in Chicago, thirty dollars in Florida supermarkets – and $9.95 in the Flower Gallery just across the street from us.

My wife said to me in the outside flower department, "Come over here and see the sick woman."

That's exactly how it sounded, amidst the racket of passing cars and trucks.

When I followed her over to the cashier's stand, I said, "I don't see any sick woman."

The cashier looked as hale and fat as the other sales clerks – who were plenty big enough.

"Sick woman?" said my wife. It was her turn to feel mystified. "What sick woman are you talking about?"

"You just said it yourself – 'Come over here and see the sick woman.' "

"I said, 'Come over here and see the cyclamen'!" She added, still annoyed, "I can understand now why so many Floridians offer to assist you in the stores. It's because you're so helpless."

"You mean, sort of a stupid shopper?"

She frowned for a moment, then sighed. "Let's just say 'helpless.' "

■■
Why Debby Boone Didn't Answer the Phone

I was watching one of those TV prank shows in Florida, and the innocent victim was Debby Boone.

At the request of the U.S. President – really a voice impersonator on the phone in the next room – she was asked to sing a terribly amateurish "new national anthem composed by the President."

Her grinning father, Pat Boone, in on the joke, stood by her shoulder as she struggled, embarrassed, through doggerel words adapted to an old English melody.

As I watched, I distinctly heard a phone ring on the TV screen.

It had no relationship to the prank.

"Somebody in that TV crew is going to catch the devil," I told myself. No doubt it hadn't been disturbing enough to warrant a retake, which might also spoil Debby's surprise.

Then it rang again. Again the performers ignored it.

"Why doesn't Debby answer that damn phone?" I asked myself, annoyed.

A blur raced past my armchair. My wife grabbed up the receiver on our sideboard phone behind me.

"Nobody there now!" she fumed.

I glanced over my shoulder. "Why should there be?"

"Because this phone has kept ringing and ringing while you sat there like a bump on a log. Are you asleep or just getting deaf?"

It had never occurred to me someone might be trying to reach us.

She stormed out of the room, glaring at me.

"I thought Debby Boone would answer the phone," I called out after her.

She put her head back in the doorway, looked at me strangely, and went on.

That's the whole trouble with TV today: the sounds are far too realistic.

Once upon a time, when I was growing up in Saint John, New Brunswick, the only sounds we usually heard were familiar and recognizable – church bells, sleigh bells, school bells, fire-wagon bells, cowbells; the fire-alarm horn, the mournful shout of the coal pedlar "C-O-A-L!", and the fish man's long-drawn holler, "Gas-per-aux!", an occasional honk from a chugging automobile, the *cling-clang* of the Italian scissors grinder as he trundled his cart along the street, the *ding-dong* of the streetcar going up a steep hill, the grunting groan of the Partridge Island fog-horn that sometimes brought a bull moose swimming out to the island hoping to find the lovesick female. And, of course, the tinkling of the little bell as you opened the door to the mom-and-pop corner grocery. (In those days fire alarms were rung by pulling down a lever in neighbourhood boxes after smashing the glass. Box Fifteen, for instance, was denoted on the city fire horn by one long blast, a brief pause, then five short blasts.)

Neither the early radios nor wind-up gramophones,

with their primitive sound reproduction, seemed very real.

Then the manufacturers began introducing lifelike technology. With diabolical ingenuity they set about driving everyone crazy.

I became aware of it one Christmas Eve when my mother came to stay.

We'd bought an electric train for our young son, and a neighbour dropped in around midnight to help me set up the tracks.

A press on a control button – and the train began to race. Rounding a curve, the locomotive blew two realistic long toots on its horn – *Whoo! Whoo!*

A hurried clatter of footsteps echoed on the upstairs landing. My mother, in a nightdress, was clutching her suitcase.

"Where's the fire?" she called down. "Did you get the number?"

Increasingly since then, I've been haunted by bells and horn blasts and other noises. My wife says I have bells in my belfry.

I can't help answering all TV show telephone rings. If I don't bother, it always turns out to be our phone.

When the TV doorbell rings repeatedly, I've learned it's hazardous to go on reading the paper and assuming it was just people winning ten-thousand-dollar prizes on a quiz program. On one occasion, not until a few moments too late did I catch a glimpse of the Reverend Mr. McFolley stomping angrily down the driveway. He'd seen me through the window, apparently reading, pretending not to hear the bell. He probably thought I was afraid he was canvassing for contributions.

Several TV game shows ring buzzers for correct or incorrect answers. I always hurry out to the kitchen stove on the chance the roast in the oven may be in danger of overcooking.

When a baby wails on our TV, I spring up out of my chair – even though our family is now grown up.

A barking dog or cat fight on TV will make me rush to the window to look.

When a siren screams, I peer out trying to see a police car or ambulance that isn't there.

A loud clap of thunder in the movie film, and I quickly disconnect the set lest a bolt of lightning blow a fuse.

If a man yells in pain, my wife's alarmed voice calls from downstairs: "Are you all right?"

Sue-Ellen on *Dallas* need only dismount from her horse, open the stable door, and shout jokingly: "Anybody home?" and my wife will shout from below, "I'm down here!"

Which, if Sue-Ellen could only hear it, would give her quite a surprise.

::

The Happy Madhouse on the Drive North

For once I realized I'm a hopelessly helpless bargain hunter. Driving back to Canada from Florida, we stopped at Freeport, Maine, to visit the legendary L.L. Bean store – the famous sportmen's and family emporium open around the clock day and night, every day of the year, including Christmas.

"So you're going to L.L. Bean's," mused the hotel desk clerk. "Your best bet would be around three o'clock in the morning. It's not so crowded then."

He didn't say whether we were supposed to get our night's sleep before, or after.

Ignoring his good counsel, we stopped in Bean's extra parking lot at ten o'clock next morning. The big country store was busy but far from jammed.

Not until we emerged did I notice the unholy bedlam coming out of what looked like a big sprawling gospel tent.

The overhead sign said: "L.L. Bean's Annual TENT SALE."

A cut-price tent would be just the thing for our younger son and his family going camping in national parks!

Squeezing my way into the mob, which was like a yard sale gone wild, I espied a large sign behind a frantic cashier:

TENT SALE
$127 for $49

Great! And well within our Canadian customs allowance.

"Where are the forty-nine-dollar tents?" I asked.

"We have no tents," said the woman.

"But your sign says tent sale and lists all the price discounts."

Said a male customer helpfully over my shoulder, "I thought it meant canoes."

"How," I persisted, "can you have a tent sale without any tents to sell?"

Explained the cashier impatiently, "The sign only means you're in a tent."

"I saw a few tents at the back," said the helpful man.

So I climbed over shoppers' feet and the good-natured backs of people trying on gumboots, and finally discovered a long box with a tent in it. I started to pull it out.

"Are you planning to climb Mount McKinley?" inquired a bystander.

"No" – in surprise – "not just now."

"Well, you're looking at a nylon backpacking tent shaped like a low igloo. It's preferred by mountaineers."

I thanked him and then started pulling from a box a voluminous blue tent in heavy folds that never seemed to end.

"Do you really know what you're looking for?" asked the man.

"No. But I thought this probably was a tent."

"I'd wait for some advice if I were you," he said. "It looks to me like you're buying a cardinal's robe."

That was the end of my tenting expedition in Freeport.

We went back into the store and bought a disposable camera for $9.95 U.S. instead. I remember it well, because the directions said, "If you find any defects, simply mail the camera back to the manufacturer and it will be repaired without charge."

The manufacturer's address was Tokyo.

The Problem of Finding New Brunswick

If we imagine that Canada's four Atlantic provinces are well known to the everyday Floridian, we're only kidding ourselves. If a Floridian has ever been to this part of Canada at all, he remembers only the lovely scenery and in New Brunswick the Magnetic Hill; in Nova Scotia, the Cabot Trail and the fact that Anne Murray came from thereabouts – conversation pieces for when he returns to the U.S.

This persistent unawareness came home to me when I visited the biggest travel agency in the St. Petersburg area, where rows of young women were arranging ticket reservations for people.

"I would like to know," I said, "what it would cost for my wife and myself to fly home to New Brunswick for Christmas."

"Let me see," said the obliging young woman, opening a big loose-leaf book. "Yes, I can get you from Tampa to New Brunswick with two changes of plane."

"One change," I interjected. "At Montreal or at Toronto or Boston."

She shook her head, and showed me the book page. *Two* changes."

"But you're looking at New Brunswick, New Jersey."

"Didn't you say you wanted to go to New Brunswick?"

"Yes, but I meant New Brunswick, Canada. It's a province of our country. You know Maine? Maine, a sort of hinterland of the United States?"

"Yes."

"Well, I want to go to New Brunswick, just beyond Maine – it's a hinterland of the hinterland."

"Where do you want to land?"

"Saint John."

She flipped the pages of another big book, stopped, and stared. Then slowly she looked up at me with the coy smile of someone who has caught a joker trying to pull her leg.

"Saint John," she said, "is in Newfoundland."

::

Amanda Hosbert's System for Beating Inflation

When I returned from the supermarket my wife said, "Your
girl-friend Amanda Hosbert stopped at the front door and
left this envelope for you. She says it contains a proven
method for senior citizens to cope with inflation, and she
knew you'd be interested."

What a relief! Old Amanda isn't even a member of the
group I call the Merry-making Widows – the ageing joke
tellers who gather on the lawn outside our back windows
and scream with laughter. But she's just as sprightly as
they are in her eighty-second year, and I think she just
loves to see my ears redden and my Adam's apple gulp
when she spins a good one.

So it was a welcome change to open the envelope and
prepare to read a scholarly treatise headed: "A SENIOR
CITIZEN BEATS INFLATION."

Here it was:

A couple aged seventy-seven went to the doctor's
office. The doctor asked, "What can I do for you?"

The man said, "Will you watch us make love?"

The doctor looked puzzled, but agreed. When the couple had finished, the doctor said, "There is nothing wrong with the way you do it." And he charged them sixteen dollars.

This happened several weeks in a row. The couple would make an appointment, have their love play, pay the doctor, and leave.

Finally the doctor asked, "Just what exactly are you trying to find out?"

The old gentleman said, "We're not trying to find out anything. She is married and we can't go to her house. I am married and we can't go to my house. Holiday Inn charges $60. Hilton charges $72. We do it here for $16 and I get back $12.80 from Medicare for a visit to the doctor's office."

That was two weeks ago, and I haven't since chanced to meet Amanda to express my thanks. It may be because I'm using the back door now.

::

It's Great To Meet Someone from Your Own Home Town!

Thousands of Canadians visiting Florida this year have been taking sea cruises from Miami and Tampa to far-away lands to add variety to their holiday experiences. They're seeing amazing sights, too.

"You should have been with me in London!" Fred Quimby exclaimed while I was waiting to be picked up at the suburban car pool. "I'll never forget it. Do you know who I saw?"

"No," I said. "Who?" I couldn't imagine, but I supposed it was Mrs. Thatcher, strolling in the park.

"Oscar Flewwelling himself!"

I couldn't place Oscar Flewwelling for a moment. Was he a great Shakespearian actor, a philosopher, or the poet laureate?

"Oh, yes," I began, "the famous . . . the famous . . ." I waited hopefully for him to finish the sentence.

"*You* know Oscar Flewwelling," Fred said a little irritably. "You've bought your groceries from him for years."

"Oh – Oscar *Flewwelling*! Sure I know him. Well, well! What do you know!"

"Yes," continued Fred enthusiastically, "I spotted him just getting on a bus at Paddington – and, boy, I had to run like blazes to catch the same bus. Gee, but it's great to meet someone from your own home town!"

"What did he say?"

"Why, nothing, really. We both just wondered what was doing back on Main Street."

"Did you see Paris?"

"*Did* I! That was the high spot of the trip! I bumped into Mrs. Birch in the Louvre – you know, the Birches on Douglas Avenue in Saint John – and then the whole Henderson family walking down the Champs Elysée. Imagine!"

"That was certainly worth going over for."

He wasn't even listening. He went on ecstatically, "And did I tell you about Pompeii? I went to see the ruins – and I saw old Miss Gribble, the school teacher from the north end, as big as life."

"Incredible!"

"Yes. I knew her right off, though I'd never met her. I introduced myself, and she said it was the most remarkable thing that happened on her whole trip."

"And what did *you* say?"

"I asked her if she knew the McGorlicks – they live in the north end, too – and she said she didn't. I said that was all right – I didn't know them, either, I just thought she might."

"Well! That was quite a coincidence, too."

"Yes, wasn't it? And I had the most astonishing experience in Venice –"

Unfortunately, then, my car came along. I've never found out to this day whom he saw in Venice, and whether they were poling a gondola or just swimming through. But it certainly must have been an astonishing sight. Europe is well worth seeing when you go to Florida.

Wives Are for Listening To

I don't know how it is with other husbands, but when I leave my wife waiting in our parked car she always thinks of a reason to call me back before I get even halfway to my destination.

It's mind-racking.

Like when I visit the bank to make a deposit.

Just as I reach the front doorway, I hear a loud honking and muffled shouts.

A dozen people turn to see what the emergency is. I hurry back and the window goes down.

"Have you got your wallet?" my wife says.

"Of course I've got my wallet."

"Then what's lying on the floor on your side? It looks like your wallet."

"You needn't have caused a commotion. I'd have realized it the minute I got into the bank."

Similarly, we go on a busy morning to the huge Orange Blossom citrus and vegetable emporium. Everyone in creation is there. Cars are darting in and backing out from all directions.

I step out to buy half a gallon of orange juice. Weaving and dodging through the confusing maze, I'm startled to hear the horn blaring short toots and see arms waving frantically to me from the car. Passing drivers stop in their tracks to stare.

I step-dance back. My wife says: "Watch those cars backing out. You nearly got run over."

"That was what I was doing–watching the cars."

"Sure! But an old nitwit woman was starting to back out right into you, and you didn't even see her."

"Well, please don't shout at me again. It gets me all rattled."

"You'd rather take the chance of getting killed?"

I sigh and think a moment, then reply, "Sometimes I wonder."

That brings us up to New Year's Eve.

We'd just returned to Seminole from a Christmas trip home to Hampton and I still had one or two presents hidden away to give my wife.

I can tell you, they were pretty special, and I had had a hard time shopping for them.

In a huge drug and discount merchandise store I asked the young manager: "Do you still have any little black ornamental tea-kettles with handles? I remember you displayed them last year, marked down from $20 to $13.75."

"Nope," he said. "I've never had any in this store."

To be absolutely positive, I asked the check-out girl, too.

"Never even seen one," she tossed off with a smile, then went right back to talking to her boy-friend on the phone. That's typical of many Florida stores. Clerks chat animatedly with each other while you wait, ignored. They don't know what the store has. Nor even what their own department has. Worse, they can't work the keys on their own sales computers.

I realized this anew when I glanced back as I was

leaving – and saw a dozen black iron ornamental kettles displayed on a sale counter for $13.95 each.

Then, having saved so much, I looked around and found another item on sale, its price cut from $22.95 to $4.95 – something that would certainly captivate any wife's heart.

It was a little machine with long tines and a handle. The idea was to press down the tine bar into the lawn with your foot, pull back the handle – and up would come the dandelion root! All you had to do then was collect the roots. I could imagine my wife having summer fun with it all day long, while I watched TV inside the house. Later she'd tell me proudly how many roots she'd pulled up.

It was a laborious job, gift-wrapping the two new presents, and I had to keep bending over to pick up stray bits of transparent tape. Every time, it seemed, since I had put on so much extra Christmas-season weight, I heard a faint sound like a thread ripping. I knew immediately it was only my old underwear. Oh, well, just five more minutes, and I'd be finished with this job, anyway.

Next day we drove two miles to our favourite service station, en route to a big department store.

"Now," I said firmly as I unbuckled my seat-belt, "are you going to yell at me when I get out?"

"No. Why should I?"

"Well, if you have anything to say, say it now. Because I am not coming back."

Still grouching, I hurriedly filled up the tank, then threaded through the crowd of motorists to pay my bill in the convenience store.

Honk! Honk! Honk! Honk!

Shaking my head, I waved the gesticulating hands away: "I'm not coming! I don't want to hear you! Tell me when I come back!"

After a few minutes of happily mingling with other

people waiting in line, I strode out of the store and climbed into our car.

"Well, now, what was all the excitement about?"

"The whole seat of your pants is open."

"What? Wide open?"

"Yes, from your crotch right up to your belt. You're a flasher from the wrong side – a rear flasher!"

"Good lord! Why didn't you tell me?"

She just looked at me, her mouth set in a firm line.

"So what do we do now?" I asked. "Can you walk into the department store right tight behind me? Or" – on a sudden impulse – "could I take off my sweater and tie its arms around my stomach and the sweater itself would cover the back view? You know, as if I was going punting on the Thames."

"We're going to drive home and I'll change your pants."

"Sh! Lord, quick, put the car window up! People will think I have a nanny."

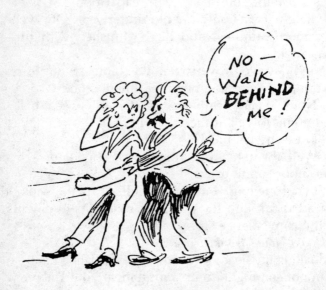

Friends who later heard about my experience were a great disappointment to me.

No one gave me the sympathy I deserved.

Almost every one, and particularly the women, said the same thing:

"That'll teach you to listen to your wife."

One Tiny Letter
Can Say a Lot

I could hardly wait to tell Amanda Hosbert, a Florida widow in her mid-eighties who lives down the street, about the strange thing that happened when I was rushed into a Clearwater hospital to have a pace-maker installed.

Amanda is a delightful person with a lively interest in everything about her. I knew she'd laugh when I showed her my souvenirs – two plastic wristbands, the kind they put on babies so the wrong mothers won't take them.

"When the nurse snipped off the first one the morning of my operation," I told Amanda, "I asked her why she was going to replace it so soon. Wasn't it just a waste of time?

"The nurse replied, 'Oh, just a slight revision.'

"So I asked her to let me compare the wristlets.

"I couldn't see any difference.

" 'Look closely,' she said. 'The first one has a capital F printed on it. The second has an M instead.'

" 'What does that mean?'

"She laughed. 'It means you were a female when you

came in yesterday, but today you're a man again.' "

That caused me to wonder momentarily: Had someone done a sex-change on me when I was sound asleep after my bedtime pill?

When my wife came in after the operation, she was no help to my morale. "Perhaps," she said, "they just took a look at your flabby chest when you were admitted."

For some reason, this upset me. I retorted angrily, "Have you never seen a Japanese wrestler?"

As I expected, kindly old Amanda laughed uproariously when I told her. Then she said, "Wait – would you like to hear my story about a ten-year-old boy?"

My spirits sank. A ten-year-old boy? I didn't want to hurt the dear old soul's feelings.

"This little boy," she said, smiling, "was always asking his grandmother to tell him her age. She kept refusing.

" 'I don't have birthdays any more,' she told him. 'So I don't know how old I am.'

"His entreaties continued without let-up.

"One day he happily announced, 'I found out how old you are! And I know all about you.'

" 'How did you find out?'

" 'I found your driver's licence in your purse. It tells everything. On the roads test it says passed.' He added sadly, 'But for sex you only got an *F*.' "

Later I said to my wife, "Why is she always telling me her sexy stories? She knows I don't want to hear them."

"Well" – my wife shrugged – "you asked for it."

The Day the Long Limousine Glided Up Our Street

"This place is dead. Nothing ever happens!" said the little lady at the end of our street in Florida.

It was dangerous talk, I knew in an instant – tempting Fate with an open invitation to liven things up, perhaps by inflicting disaster on our tranquil row of town houses.

My foreboding didn't have long to wait.

I was just stepping into the shower next morning when my wife shouted through the door: "Are we on fire?"

Dashing out, with my dressing-gown hurriedly tied, I heard sirens wailing everywhere.

On the street was a huge red fire truck, throbbing loudly, with a crew of men rushing about in full regalia, ready to face any crisis. Voices were barking commands over two-way speakers.

Spectators – some dressed and some of the women in negligés or housecoats – were hurrying past us and heading down the street. Across from the lady's home, smoke was coming from the roof and blowing into the apartment. More fire trucks were on the scene there, and also a rescue van – a sight worthy of a TV news clip.

Then the word filtered up the sidewalk grapevine –
"Just a short circuit in the air conditioning. Nobody hurt.
No damage."

At least it probably taught that lively little lady what
careless talk can do.

Nobody was hurt, I stated – except perhaps my own
feelings.

I said good morning to a woman standing out in her
negligé watching the activity. She just frowned at me.

"Odd," I said to my wife. "I've often talked with her
up at the mailbox."

"She's short-sighted. She doesn't know you. She thinks
you're one of the women in housecoats."

"With a moustache?"

"She can't see it."

Then, to make it worse, my wife called out in panic to
me, a few steps ahead:

"Quick! Pull down your dress in the back!" My thin
cotton robe had got caught up in its belt in the back.

"That's terrible!" I said when we got into our apartment. "You said 'dress' – it's a *dressing*-gown. Now that
woman will be sure you're living with a female who has
a moustache."

But the very next day I discovered a vengeful Fate
wasn't finished with our street yet.

Moving slowly up the other side purred a beautiful
long pearl-grey limousine – just like the stretched-out
models the mob godfathers use in New York. But this
one had tasselled curtains and ornate silver ornamenta-
tion towards the rear.

"Oh, lord," my wife exclaimed, "a hearse! Who's it
for?"

Strangely, when there's a fire everyone rushes out into
the street to see. When it's a hearse, people stay indoors,
jostling each other for the best viewing spot through the
curtains in the kitchen window.

The hearse stopped. The driver stepped out with a big pad under his arm, and looked at the house number.

"Heavens," my wife said: "I hope it's not the Kamenskis. She's been looking pale. Poor old fellow, he couldn't get along without her."

But the driver walked on to the next house and stared up again.

"Mrs. McGoligan!" my wife said. "Oh, I hope not. She was always a lovely person."

This door-by-door procedure kept up until the driver reached a house on the end of the short block. He checked the street number, rang the bell, and was admitted.

We waited, holding our breath.

A few minutes later the door re-opened. Out came the driver, heading back towards the hearse – followed by an attractive middle-aged woman in a bright pink jogging outfit.

I was dumbfounded.

"Is this the new self-serve?" I asked my wife. "Does the modern corpse walk to the hearse?"

But they strolled right by it, and the man started to examine minutely the lady's own car, a big beautiful antique Cadillac.

When I sauntered past, trying to look uninterested, I realized she was only having it appraised for sale. The man was a dealer. The hearse itself, to my surprise, had whitewash lettering on a side window: "FOR SALE – $2,500." Underneath was the phone number to call.

Excited, I told my wife, "Imagine – that wonderful limousine for only $2,500! I'd love to buy it and drive it back to Canada."

She looked at me coldly: "Why?"

"Such a bargain! And any young person, like our grandson in Fredericton, would love it!"

"Don't be ridiculous. Everyone would stare at you. In Saint John traffic would stop and men would tip their hats."

"No – I'd put a big sign on the side: TENNESSEE MOUNTAIN CLOG-DANCERS TROUPE."

"Stop talking about it. You haven't got $2,500 anyway."

"But I'd love to drive in that limousine."

"Forget it. You'll be driving in one soon enough."

Real Estate Fast Talkers? We Showed Florida How

Hearing about the unending procession of Florida real estate developers, bankers, politicians, judges, and others wending its melancholy way to the courts, I can't help thinking that we in Atlantic Canada had the best wheeler-dealer of them all. The story could have happened in Florida today.

Every community should have a booster like Jim Adverse. I'll never forget what he did for Shadydale, a little suburb I lived in each summer to get away from the city.

For many years Shadydale dozed under the pines beside the St. John River. Every day the town's two dozen families took basket lunches to the beach. The kids played in the water, the mothers knitted and talked, the fathers fly-fished for the Atlantic silver salmon they imagined were lurking in the ripply water off the sand-bar. In their ignorance they thought they were having a wonderful time.

That's how Shadydale was when Jim Adverse rented a cottage. It never was the same again.

Jim immediately realized the place was not progressive; it had no community spirit. He had quite a reputation as a go-getter in the city, a regular human dynamo, and he knew what he was talking about.

When he pointed out that not one new cottage had been built in eight years, we could only hang our heads. It was the truth.

"If we're not going forwards," Jim said, "we're going backwards. There's no such thing as standing still."

We could not dispute that.

"So we've got to work together to develop Shadydale," Jim went on. "We've got to grow. Progress must be our watchword!"

We cheered him to a man, thankful that destiny had sent us someone in time.

Jim organized the Shadydale Awake committee, and we put aside our salmon rods to attend meetings every day. By passing the hat we raised money to advertise Shadydale in the city papers as the last unspoiled resort on the river.

The results exceeded our fondest hopes. New families flocked in, and cottages sprang up like mushrooms. Everybody sold his flower garden for a hundred dollars to make another building lot, and we chipped in and bought Jim Adverse a gold watch because progress was making us rich.

Naturally the beach became crowded, so we dredged out swamp land to enlarge it, assessing ourselves a hundred dollars apiece to pay for the job. This attracted more homes, crowding the beach again.

So many new faces appeared that the girls were nervous about walking the paths at night; accordingly we taxed ourselves to bring in electric lights, and the new power station took over the salmon rapids.

The lighted paths drew throngs of walkers, making the gravel lanes a quagmire in wet weather; we hoisted our taxes to asphalt the roads and bypaths.

You never saw such progress—steamrollers, hot tar,

power linesmen, carpenters, bricklayers. Jim Adverse said we were witnessing the birth of a township, and we were so thrilled we notched up our taxes to present him with the cottage he had rented. It was the least we could do, we told him, and he agreed.

Our property taxes were now 12 per cent per year — but Jim assured us a community had to spend money to make money, which was only common sense.

The resort got so thickly settled the wells were condemned, and we installed a water and sewage system. Jim arranged this so it didn't cost us a cent; we just floated a bond issue, selling the bonds to ourselves. We floated another when people began to winterize their cottages and demanded a fine school of which Shadydale could be proud.

We carried Jim Adverse on our shoulders the day the news came that Shadydale had been acclaimed "North America's most progressive community." This certainly made up for the fact that it also had North America's most progressive tax rate.

All the pine trees had to be chopped down to clear the approaches for our new airport. We didn't mind, after Jim pointed out that nature couldn't stand in the way of progress. Besides, the new one-man sawmill down by the power station needed the trees to make lumber, so it was a matter of saving a home industry and preventing unemployment.

When the airport came in, of course, the name "Shadydale" had to go. The Shadydale Awake committee said it sounded like a hamlet. The chamber of commerce complained that too much mail was arriving addressed to Shady Deal, which was bad for business. The church ladies' auxiliary threw its full weight into the agitation right after the annual chicken and strawberry pie dinner, passing a resolution that as the pines were gone there was no shade now anyway, and the old name collapsed under the strain.

They renamed it Adverse City.

With the roar of planes, the racket from the sawmill, the smoke from the power station, it had become more like a city than my home town; and there was no point to moving from one city to another city every summer. So I moved my family five miles up the river to a tranquil little birch-shaded resort known as Happy Acres.

Soon afterwards I learned that Adverse City's tax rate, progressing anew with the cost of the police department, the new tax office building, and the new civic garbage collection system, had reached 100 per cent. Jim Adverse packed up and left, saying his work was done.

They held a banquet for him. Speakers wept openly when they said if it hadn't been for Jim they wouldn't have had an attractive public building like the tax office because there would have been no taxes to collect; no superb modern police department, because the former residents were too peaceful to need one; and no garbage collection system, because they hadn't thought of garbage until they met him.

The city gave him a gold key to Adverse City, and he gave the city back his house, which just exactly paid for last year's taxes on it.

Before Jim managed to get away from the banquet, the chief tax collector passed him a note to remind him that he had lived in Adverse City for four months and one week of the current year also; so Jim wrapped the gold key in his paper napkin, with the gold watch, and slipped it to him under the table.

I heard the other day that Jim Adverse has been seen walking around Happy Acres, looking for a cottage to rent and musing that the birch trees would make great hardwood flooring if someone had the initiative to build a planing mill. Other than one case of scarlet fever, that's the only bad news the place has had since we came.

I'm Right in Tune with All the Old Songs

'm glad the old songs are coming back. They make me young again.

Formerly when I sat in a restaurant at noon quietly humming, "You're the Cream in My Coffee" or "That's My Weakness Now," I'd stop dead when I suddenly realized the waitresses were tittering, and people were looking at me with the curiosity due an aged Elizabethan minstrel who had wandered in and started playing madrigals on his lute.

Today, when I hum the same tunes, they listen admiringly. I overhear a waitress saying, "That's the song I was telling you about, the one that advertises Blemish-Ban on TV. I wish I knew what it's called." On this cue I hum "Chloe," and a little more loudly, keeping time unconcernedly with the tines of the fork on the butter dish, so they'll know here's a fellow who keeps right up with the latest on TV; or, better still, they may speculate I have something to do with making commercials and I'm just in town on a vacation trip, looking for new talent.

Yes, the old songs are wonderful. But I live in dread

of someone in the family liking an old ballad on the radio when I'm not around. They never seem to hear the name; they just catch a few notes of the chorus. Then they train me to memorize it and hum the notes for the man in the music store, so I can bring home the cussed cassette the next day.

There are always a few people – usually smirky young people – loitering inside the little music store when I get there. This has happened so often it can't be passed off as mere coincidence. They're waiting for me to come in and make a fool of myself.

They pretend to be rummaging through stacks of sheet music for a special song, which they never find, or running a finger down a list of recordings. But I can feel them watching me out of the corners of their eyes, and when I turn my back to speak to the proprietor I can almost hear the exchange of knowing winks, for the fun is about to begin.

The proprietor, Mr. Gullwhistle, seems to be smiling a little too good-humoredly when he greets me. He rubs his hands with what looks very much like gleeful anticipation. This is the kind of thing that brightens up his day.

"Yes?" he says, "and what can I do for you?"

"Oh, it's nothing really important," I explain with what is meant to be a carefree grin, as though I just happened to be in a devil-may-care mood when I was passing his door. "I thought you might possibly have a cassette of a tune I heard on the air."

"Sure. Wassa name?"

"We didn't quite get the name. But the chorus went something like this" – here I draw a deep breath and lower my voice confidentially – "dee, dee, di, di, di, di, dum."

An awkward pause. All five "customers" in the store have been waiting for this moment, and they're watching Mr. Gullwhistle's face expectantly. He is frowning slightly at me, pretending to be oblivious of the gallery, but I feel sure I can detect a trace of amusement playing about his mouth.

"I don't recognize it," he says finally. "Which is funny, because I keep up with all the new hits. You sure you got it right?"

"Well, yes, pretty sure. It has a nice swing to it." Here I look absent-mindedly at the wall, at a calendar picture of a girl whose dog's leash has got tangled with her knees, as so easily happens to girls on wall calendars, and I repeat the notes softly: "Dee, dee, di, di, di, dum . . ." I have to do this abstractedly because he didn't actually ask me for an encore. The purpose is to jog his memory in case the second rendering may strike a responsive chord and he will exclaim, "Why, of course – 'I Wonder Who's Kissing Her Now.'"

If this were only a movie scene, I tell myself, all I would need to do is sing the first three or four notes – and the music store proprietor would echo the same bar in counter-harmony, and the man thumbing through the song sheets would slip over to the piano and begin playing the ac-companiment, and the young fellow scanning the record list would pluck a bass viol out of nowhere, and the other customers would suddenly be blowing clarinets and trumpets, and the music would be swelling up and filling the theatre.

But this isn't a movie. It only shows things don't always work out so well in real life.

Mr. Gullwhistle is now eyeing me with a patient tol-erance that borders on contempt. He has to. It would be serious for him to admit, in front of all these customers, that: (1) he can't recognize tunes anyway; or (2) his store doesn't have many of the newer records. He has no choice but to discredit my ear for music.

"If I were you," he suggests gently, "I would wait until I heard it on the radio again. Then I would try to pick it out on the piano right away and write a memo of the notes for me."

In embarrassment I accept this advice gratefully, hastening to point out that I was only half listening to the radio at the time anyhow; and besides, getting the cassette isn't important. As I said before, it was just a notion I had as I was walking past the store.

Now that we have both agreed I'm musically irresponsible, I take advantage of the opening to make a third and last desperate try. I shake my head good-naturedly and in apparent self-derision I say, "Isn't it strange! I could have taken my oath that the chorus went: Dee, dee, di, di, di, di, dum. . . ."

Mr. Gullwhistle shakes his head, too. "If I didn't know better," he says, "I could swear it was a bar from 'The Star Spangled Banner.'"

"That's what I would have said if you'd asked me," exclaims the young man who is poring over the list of cassettes. As a matter of fact, no one has asked him anything, and I wish he would kindly get on with his business and stop trying to impress Mr. Gullwhistle by admiring his quick perception and associating himself with it.

"I do remember," I remark hopelessly as I turn to leave, "that the words 'June star' were in it somewhere."

"Won't you come dance on the window sill, my lovely?" says Mr. Gullwhistle suddenly.

This is ridiculous, I know immediately. He is only quoting a lyric from a song, because this store doesn't have a window sill, so I stand my ground. He goes on:

". . . dance on the window sill, my lovely, my June star twinkling in the midnight blue . . . dee, dee, di, di, di, di, dum. . . ."

"There! That's it! That's the tune I was singing!"

"Now, now. You were singing di, di, di, dum, dum, di. It's a real oldie, but it's coming back big on TV ads, I understand."

"Well, I certainly thought I –"

"If you want my opinion," intercedes the cassette-hunting customer, not waiting to see whether anyone does, "you were singing di, di, di, dum, dum, di. Mr. Gullwhistle is right." On saying this he smiles ingratiatingly at the proprietor, and I don't doubt he is working his way up to ask, after I've been got rid of, whether he can take home a few cassettes just to try out for the weekend.

I have no alternative but to pay Mr. Gullwhistle and leave with my hard-won recording under my arm, thinking dark thoughts about young foot-kissing creeps so unprincipled as to chime in with someone else's utterly wrong argument.

Some day I would like to be back in that store, merely browsing around, when that same smarty-pants wimp comes in asking for a recording of an old-time hit which his girl-friend has just heard on the radio but whose name he can't recall. Mr. Gullwhistle will be mystified, but I will understand immediately that the fellow is trying to hum "Dardanela," a Guy Lombardo version of which is on the display shelf right beside his ear.

It will give me great pleasure, despite my own high principles, to agree readily with Mr. Gullwhistle that if we didn't know different we'd swear he was humming "Columbia the Gem of the Ocean." And we will stare the young man out of the place, and chuckle uproariously to ourselves.

My Venture into International Finance

It came as a complete surprise when I returned from Florida. I opened a long envelope from Iowa, and out popped a cheque for one dollar – an American dollar!

I was mystified. Did I know anyone in Clinton, Iowa? Who could my benefactor be?

Then I remembered. When I was in Florida a Toronto friend planning to leave on a tour of the Orient told me, "I have a dollar rebate slip for wine to send in. I'll put your name and address here on it, and you're welcome to it, because we'll be gone."

"Let me give you the postage anyway." I laughed, insisting he accept a U.S. twenty-five-cent stamp.

This daily flood of rebate letters, millions of them, I'm certain, is what keeps the U.S. post office alive.

"Well," I thought, looking at the cheque, "it's only a dollar. But a dollar is a dollar."

I drove to my bank and offered the signed cheque to the young woman teller.

"I'd like to cash this U.S. one-dollar cheque, please."

"Yes," she said, "that is one dollar."

"That's what I said, it's one dollar. I want to cash it."

"Our charge on U.S. cheques is one dollar."

"You mean it will cost me a dollar to get a dollar?"

"That's right, unless it's a U.S. Treasury cheque. Is it a Treasury cheque?"

"Well, not exactly. It's from the Almaden Wine Company. You see, a friend of mine in Florida bought a three-litre jug for $4.99 U.S. plus 6 per cent tax. He thought it would make the price even lower by sending in the rebate slip, and he put my name and address on it."

"At least you'll get the exchange on the dollar," she said.

"How much is that? The 25$^{1}/_{4}$ cents I see marked on your sign?"

"No, that's if you're buying American money. When you're selling, the exchange will give you 21$^{1}/_{2}$ cents."

"But I've already spent 30 cents U.S. for an American stamp. That's 37 cents Canadian. So I'll really get just $1.21.5 minus 37 cents – that's 84$^{1}/_{2}$ cents – and you want a dollar out of it."

"That's right."

"So I'll really get nothing."

"Well, you'll be out only a few cents."

She was trying to be helpful. "If you had a chequing account in Florida, you could mail it to them. Of course the postage would cost forty-three cents."

"But I'd be ashamed to send a deposit of only one dollar. And if I sent more with it, I'd have to pay today's exchange rate for the extra."

A happy thought struck me: I could take it down to Florida next winter, and at the bank say just casually: "Oh, what's this in my pocket? Ha! Ha! Only a dollar cheque. But I suppose I might as well cash it."

I explained this to the young woman and I said, "Isn't that a good idea?"

"Yes," she replied. "When was the cheque made out?"

"Around May, I imagine. It went to my address in Florida, and was forwarded to me here."

"It may be outdated when you get there. Many cheques are valid for only six months."

That's how matters stand as of now.

I haven't mentioned the conversation with the teller to my wife, who likes to remind me that every time I go to the bank I use another fifty cents' worth of gas. A dollar, after all, is too small an amount to burden a busy wife with.

So you'll be seeing a framed one-dollar cheque on the wall over my typewriter, and people will say, "Look – he's never cashed it. Money means nothing to him."

Which, in this case, is correct.

■■
A Visit from "The Girls" Always Baffles Me

In Canada just as in the United States, I hear, the chummy "first-name" trend is growing steadily. Down here in Florida, store clerks, doctors' receptionists, telephone canvassers, even bank accountants tell you blithely, "I'm Shana – just ask for Shana when you call back."

A Saint John, New Brunswick, woman, returning from a reunion of her nursing graduation class in Montreal, told me, "I was astonished! Years ago we nurses were always called Miss Smith, Miss Jones, Miss Brown, and so on. Now it's just Susan and Cecily and Tanya – everyone goes by her first name. They claim patients feel more at home in the friendly casual atmosphere. I think it's terrible – a professional nurse deserves more respect."

My wife, who trained earlier at another large Montreal hospital, seemed horrified, too. In her years there, she recalled, nurses called each other only by their bare surnames. Often they didn't even know their friends' first names.

That's why even today when some of her old classmates come visiting us in Florida and the doorbell rings, she calls out from the shower, "Will you answer it? It's probably Weatherby, Johnston, Green, and O'Gaffigan."

I expect to see a firm of lawyers march in carrying briefcases. But it's just four of "the girls," as she calls them, who graduated with her.

Instead of the solemn legal faces I anticipated, there's shrieking and laughter and gossip and twittering chatter. One of the girls, still breathless, turns to me:

"Where's Stiles?"

Stiles? I have to think, frowning, for a moment.

Then I realize they mean my wife.

"Oh! Mildred's in the shower. She'll be right here."

I can't feel comfortable, somehow, hearing these grown women referred to as "the girls." But then I remember I still refer to my high-school classmates, when we get together rarely, as "the boys." Old friends, in our minds, never get any older.

But times are certainly changing – fast – towards informality. The last time I was in the Saint John Regional Hospital for several days I found it sometimes difficult to figure out who was who. Not only had many of the traditional white caps disappeared, but an occasional nurse didn't even wear a gold pin or any other identification.

"You've seen that on TV hospital series," my wife reminded me. "It just never registered on you before."

I dread to think that, as the informal trend spreads, the resident doctor next time may tell me casually, " 'Old Knifer' will be here soon – he's your surgeon."

For some reason I'll expect to see a brawny, hairy-chested, swaggering character with a sport shirt wide open down to his belt, chomping on a cigar. But doubtless he will look very normal, even mild-natured, when he walks in.

"You're going to operate on me?" I'll ask hopefully.

"Yes, but I don't know for sure. It may be 'Shaky Fingers.' "

That's great. I hope I'm under the anaesthetic before Shaky Fingers appears. And I hope I come out of it again.

Late one evening, facing tests the next morning, I began to wonder anxiously if the staff was remembering my schedule. When I saw an attractive young woman in a trim white pants suit starting to pass my door I called to her:

"I'm due for my third dose of Epsom salts."

She paused and looked in.

"That's interesting." She smiled. "I'm a visitor from Bangor, Maine. I came to see my great-aunt."

No wonder she smiled. But, after all, she had no business going around looking like a nurse.

Hit the Old Spoil-sport Again, Gang!

I don't know why, but Fate has ordained that I shall take endless punishment at parties – particularly at get-togethers of Canadian winter residents and their uninhibited American friends. Both countries try to outdo each other in sheer exuberance.

I'm thumped mercilessly on the back by people for no offence other than that they remember they went to grade four with me. I'm jabbed sharply in the ribs by people who tell jokes; otherwise, they fear, I won't know when they come to the good parts. I'm pounded heartily in the stomach by people who ask why I don't take off weight, evidently under the impression that it can be punched off.

Especially am I punished for not looking happy enough. This, I have learned, is the most heinous crime that can be committed at a high-spirited social gathering, and it arouses the immediate general indignation it deserves.

Goodness knows, the guests do all they can to help me. They toot horns in my ear, throw streamers at my face, stuff confetti down my neck, blow paper gadgets that unreel out to a feather tip and knock my eye glasses askew. And yet, they say in pained puzzlement, I don't laugh; I just look rattled.

As the evening wears on, I'm certain to be hit over the head with a table dictionary by a hilarious woman with a glass in her other hand, who wants to know what's the matter with me. The theory is that this will cure me. "Smile! Smile! Smile!" she screams merrily, whacking me at every word while eager onlookers urge her on to "Sock him again—*make* him smile."

When she tires out, it doesn't stop. Other party goers jump in gladly to shake my shoulders, twist my nose, pummel my lapels. They gleefully grab my tie and yank it tight on the chance that strangulation will work as a last resort.

They had high hopes for me, I'm told, the night they persuaded a retired RCMP judo instructor and his Lionel Strongfort friend from Wisconsin to sneak up from behind and give me an airplane spin, followed by bouncing me off the wall and clamping a hammer-lock on me.

Everyone shrieked with mirth. They expected me to die laughing; I expected merely to die. When I came out of it looking no happier than before, they unanimously agreed there wasn't a spark of fun in me.

I'm sure I *would* look happier if I could just get in a few blows myself, but I have found that for some reason most people pretend to be surprised and even angry when you hit them back. And I have no intention of hitting the judo instructor.

My inability to get into the proper spirit of things worries me greatly, which makes me look less happy at each party. This compels my friends to redouble their exertions to bring me out of it. I hear they are planning to toss me into the lake at the next one.

■■
My Big Bargain!

I'm tired of hearing New Brunswick vacationers here boasting they can get four pounds of margarine in supermarkets for as little as $1.00 U.S.

Talk about bargains–I'm the real expert! I find these and better ones every day.

For instance, I read in the home newspapers and I heard on News of Canada radio here that the Bank of Canada had hit upon an ingenious idea to use up its overstock of Canadian one-dollar bills. This idea would pave the way to force everyone to use the controversial one-dollar coins called "loonies."

The plan: offer forty one-dollar greenbacks in uncut sheets to anyone who wanted to buy them as an interesting novelty to frame or as a collector's item.

If the public responded readily, the bills would soon vanish, people would get accustomed faster to the loonies, and Canada would not face the embarrassment the United States did when people rejected the Susan B. Anthony dollar coin, tens of millions of which are still piled up in federal repositories.

At Christmas time I mailed in my forty-dollar cheque from Hampton. After all, the sheet might be worth forty-five dollars in a few years.

Of course, you never know for sure about these things. I remember long ago saving fifty "Mountie" quarters and ten years later, taking them with high anticipation to show a coin dealer.

"What are they worth now?" I asked eagerly.

He looked up at me with sad patience: "Twenty-five cents apiece."

Last week a reply came from the Bank of Canada, Ottawa – with my cheque enclosed:

> We are returning your one-dollar bank-note request for the following reasons:
>
> (1) Insufficient funds. Fifty-dollar charge per sheet.
> (2) Provincial sales tax required.
> (3) Registered mail fee required.
> (4) Certified cheque or money order required.
> (5) Remittance is to be made payable to the Bank of Canada.

Anyone who thought he was helping a hapless Ottawa get rid of dollar bills received a shock – the federal government was trying to make its money make money. In short, helping itself.

The nabobs of the Bank of Canada were telling the people: "If you want to change forty dollars into forty one-dollar bills, it will cost you fifty dollars.

But the real shocker was to see they demanded that I pay provincial sales tax on the transaction, just as though they were selling me a TV set or a new carpet.

So a New Brunswicker, with an 11 per cent sales tax, would pay the Bank of Canada at least fifty-six dollars for forty dollars, not counting the registered mail fee.

It might even become a bargain if enough time went by – say, fifty years – but as I don't expect to be waiting in the wings by then, just wearing them, I'm forgoing the opportunity.

But what will come next?

Meanwhile, no one should tell Ottawa about the plan that was discussed in Washington recently to tax everyone a small percentage on his savings deposits as he made them at the bank.

Is There Really a Florida "Lucky Food"?

Canadians spending the holiday season among Florida friends would do well to familiarize themselves first with the dishes the natives enjoy. Or they'll be in for some shocks.

Personally, I've tried shark steak (far too rich) but balked at trying catfish, frog's legs, and big shrimp with the hard-crusted tails, which remind me of chicken feet.

However, Floridians flinch when I say I enjoy the purplish seaweed we eastern Canadians call dulse, and tell them, "Just give me a bent pin and I'll finish off a whole pound of fresh-cooked periwinkles (sea snails)."

So I wondered what I was in for when our merry-hearted neighbour Vera, a maiden lady, said before New Year's she was going to bring me a special "health and wealth treat" to start off the New Year auspiciously – "a great Southern tradition."

Somehow I got the idea that the awesome test of swallowing Vera's special concoction would not arise for several merciful weeks, because she said, "I always like to have corn bread, too, and I've been unable to get one of the essential ingredients, cracklin's – crisp-browned hog skin – to give flavour to the corn bread.''

Lord! Browned hog skins!

But, sure enough, at noon on New Year's Day, a beaming Vera appeared at our apartment door carrying a bowl covered with aluminum foil.

"Happy New Year!" she exclaimed. "Here's your treat – hog jowls and black-eyed peas, hot and ready to eat. Good health and good fortune to you both!"

I thanked her and wished her a Happy New Year, too.

Now, as everyone knows, people are apt to stay up pretty late to celebrate New Year's Eve. And a great many don't feel like eating anything at all by noon the next day, let alone hot hog jowls.

I gingerly lifted the shiny foil off, and you know, I had to admit it didn't appear so bad – like ham in a stew. It resembled long shredded pieces of New Brunswick baked ham in a bean soup.

But I kept staring, shaking my head, thinking of those words: "hog jowls."

"It's only ham," my wife gently reminded me. "If they called butt ham 'hog's buttocks,' you wouldn't try it, either."

Resolutely I dipped up a spoonful and tasted it.

It was delicious. I took a few more spoonfuls. My wife had some, too.

Next noon, January 2, I ate the rest of the dishful, and went next door to tell Vera how good it was.

"I just finished it," I said cheerfully.

Her face fell. "You didn't have any on New Year's Day?"

"Oh, yes, I enjoyed it then, too."

"Thank goodness," she sighed. "That was your good-luck day – New Year's Day!"

It made me smile at the superstitiousness of some people. Fortunately, I'm not credulous myself at all. That is, of course, unless you want to be ridiculous enough to count the fact that I couldn't turn on the TV to watch the Tampa Bay Buccaneers when they got into the National Football League play-offs. You see, the first three times I tuned in to a game after arriving in Florida, the quarterback immediately tossed the football right into the hands of an opposing player. So, much as I wanted to see the final games, I decided to do Tampa Bay a favour by not watching them. I just read the paper and waited for Vera to come to the door and say who won.

A thought-provoking thing happened a couple of days after New Year's. A housewife who resides on the same floor came in to see the handmade ornaments from New Brunswick on our Christmas tree before we took it down. I told her half-jokingly about the good-luck superstition of hog jowls and black-eyed peas.

"Oh, it's very true!" she said, suddenly serious. "Why, two years ago Vera brought us a bowl. It was very tasty – and in the following year our family business met with phenomenal success. The next New Year's she brought us another dish – and we had another outstanding year.

"Naturally, this time I asked her early for the good-luck dish, but I was really worried when New Year's Day came and we hadn't heard from her. Then the phone rang, and Vera said, 'Shank yourself down here quick – I've got your hog jowls and black-eyed peas ready.' Was I ever relieved to start the New Year right!"

And Vera started it right, too. She assured me so herself. That same day she fell backwards into her clothes closet and banged herself up so badly she had to spend six weeks in hospital.

"Am I ever lucky!" she exclaimed when she got out. "Phoebe Haskell fell that very day, and she hadn't had hog jowls and black-eyed peas. She's still all strung up in a hospital bed."

▪▪ Florida's Style Parade: Something Old, But New Again

By now you've undoubtedly felt aghast at the bizarre new styles created by the couturiers of famed French, Italian, and British salons. Some models exhibit Oriental pantaloons as blown up as the clothes of Tweedledum and Tweedledee. Big-brimmed hats are back. Mink and other furs are displayed in short jackets and long coats.

But you'll see an even more spectacular parade here in Florida when a cold or rainy spell hits for two or three days about once every winter. If the thermometer falls to freezing at 4:00 A.M., and only gets up to fifty-five degress Fahrenheit at noon, the residents think this surely must be what life in Alaska is like. They walk along the streets a little bent over and hugging themselves.

Women wear short wool skirts (which they'd put away in 1930) over jogging pants. On their heads are slightly threadbare fur hats, relics of their younger days in Minnesota, Wisconsin, or Toronto, or toques or tams or wool scarves; on their feet, snow boots, heavy joggers, or a style of boot with high, square-cut heels which my wife calls "clunkers" – popular twenty-five years ago. And they wear old wool gloves that show there are moths in Florida, too.

The big enclosed shopping malls and the one-dollar movie houses are thronged with patrons glad to get out of the cold (and sneakily calculating how much they'll save on their home heating system for three hours).

People in discount department stores sneeze freely over you and mutter, "Isn't the flu God-awful this year? They say the snow-birds brought it down." (Snow-brids are anyone in the upper U.S. snow zone, also all the Canadians.)

Everyone watches TV weather predictions – often wrong – to know whether to cover their perishable plants outdoors. Nobody, if it's a dry winter, is allowed to hose his flowers, shrubs, lawn, or car in the daytime hours.

They're scared stiff, as consumers, to hear that the widespread crop losses will soon send the prices of tomatoes and other fresh vegetables, including strawberries, sky-high.

People read with apprehension of the rapid spread of "wildfires," the Florida name for forest fires. Paradoxically, they're fought with "fire bombs" to contain their advance.

But even more terrifying to some is the imminent peril of sink-holes, which can suddenly swallow up a few cars or a house at one gulp. Apparently they are caused by resources that are drawn nearly dry by the constant hosing of the strawberry groves to encase the berries in ice – which, extraordinarily, keeps them from freezing. Meanwhile, the water from the spraying is overloading the ground.

However, after all the scares in the headlines about sink-holes, only a handful occur, one engulfing an unoccupied outbuilding of a school; a doctor diagnosing the phenomenon from across the street said, "I am not worried. I feel that the Lord has always been with me, and will stay with me." As I pen these words, the Lord apparently is still with him. And the doctor is still with us.

Meanwhile, as always, warm sunny weather returns, for the time being, at least. The American Automobile Association emergency crews in St. Petersburg, who had answered hundreds of calls for two mornings to jump start balky cars, are able to take a restful snooze, just like the Maytag repairman on TV.

And to my surprise the annual strawberry festival turns out to be the biggest ever, with half a million pints of luscious berries served on shortcakes or sold outright. Luxuriant plenty despite TV panoramas of scorched-out strawberry fields!

And what of all the hullabaloo about food prices going through the ceiling?

We've been told that the cold spell and high winds were disastrous to northern and central Florida's leading farm products – tomatoes, peppers, squash, corn, potatoes, cucumbers, beans, lettuce, celery, radishes, and carrots. But we have to remember the resourcefulness of Florida's food brokers, who in a flash can bring in provisions from other parts of the United States and Central America. And remember, too, that in this sunny climate second plantings will come along very swiftly.

You hear many people telling each other, "This was the worst winter freeze in Florida's history."

Nonsense.

A chilly interlude comes every January or February.

I remember one winter when a skim of snow appeared, and school kids wearing socks on their hands insteads of mitts, were yelling with glee as they hurled snowballs at each other. That was a year some big department stores found it impossible to heat the buildings sufficiently, and all the clerks wore their coats.

And Sally, the plump old maid at a checkout, announced loudly, "Cripes, I was so freezing in bed last night I wished to God for once I'd got married."

My Keep-Young Formula Worked on Howard

I always thought if someone my age lived in a quiet town-house development among folks five or ten years older, he'd feel like a spry young fellow by comparison.

It doesn't seem to work that way.

My eighty-two-year-old Seminole neighbour, from Regina, is a sad illustration.

Heaven knows, I tried hard to buoy up Howard McKendrill's outlook.

It was a hopeless task.

"Everything's so silent here I can't sleep," he complained. "When I hear a siren in the dead of night, it's never a good fire I can go out and watch. It's the ambulance."

He went on disconsolately, "If I hear a clanking racket outside our door in the morning, it isn't a happy gardener going by with his wheelbarrow; it's an old fellow pushing a walker. I can't go out and compare ailments with these people, because I've got nothing to compare."

"But one good thing," I countered, "is every day the

St. Petersburg newspaper prints a couple of dispatches about wonderful new cures discovered for senior citizens' ailments. Like psyphoplenoxis – doctors say we'll be completely free of it in thirty years! Of course, you don't have it anyway."

"I'm not sure," he replied. "But if I did, then I wouldn't be rid of it until I reached 103."

You see? It's just impossible to comfort some people.

"What are the symptoms?" he asked suddenly.

"A sharp pain in both feet when you wake up in the morning. It fades out after a few minutes of walking."

"Good God – I already have it! I had it even before the newspaper heard about it. Is it dangerous?"

"Well, I don't think it's fatal," I told him with a smile, "because I just realized I've had it myself for the last three years."

He didn't laugh. He only looked straight ahead, frowning.

Seizing on a new approach, I reminded him cheerily, "You don't even have any aches or pains, which is remarkable. You're very lucky. Remember the doctors' old-time saying, 'If you're past seventy and you wake up in the morning with no pains, you're dead!"

For some reason again he didn't smile. I just couldn't figure the fellow out.

Jokingly again, I advised him, "Heck, pay no attention to those doctors! Why, every time they announce two new cures, then they report they've discovered four brand-new diseases."

Howard shook his head. "That's the whole trouble. Everybody in our condominium is already sick; it's not fair to expect them to take on new ailments."

At this point I decided to have a talk with Sybil, Howard's well-meaning wife.

"I was going to raise his spirits by remarking we're getting fewer phone calls from cemetery hucksters this winter," I told her. "I think the Garden of Blessed Remembrance Advance Niche Payment Plan has given up on me after eighteen winters. I'm a great disappointment to them."

She sighed. "It wouldn't do any good. He's convinced that Florida doesn't add ten years to his life, as they always say; he thinks it only adds ten years to his age. He just sits and watches TV and waits for the end.

"Even then he isn't happy. He's driven crazy by the continual commercials about how senior citizens can get insurance for final expenses for only $4.95 to $6.50 a month. He shouts back angrily at our TV because the commentators – Glenn Ford, Art Linkletter, Danny Thomas, Ed McMahon, and a dozen more – rarely hint how much coverage you get for that."

"He should look at the brighter side," I said. "It's a laugh how most of those pitch men wear old men's homey coat sweaters and open-necked shirts to show they're just ordinary folks themselves."

Then, out of a clear blue Florida sky, the inspiration hit me.

"Why not take him down to that famous Coliseum ballroom where the big bands play? Get him exercising, dancing! Mixing with young fry! He'd feel the years drop away."

To my surprise, she actually did.

I happened to be walking past when they drove home at 11:30.

"Well!" I enthused. "How'd you enjoy it? Aren't you back early?"

Howard's face inside the car looked glum. I could see I'd failed again.

"Took a cramp in my right leg," he said. "The only ones I danced with anyway were Sybil and some skinny maiden ladies older than us."

Crawling out of the car, he took a cramp again and tumbled to the sidewalk. I helped Sybil get him into the apartment.

Next afternoon I knocked on his door. I braced myself for the bawling out.

"Oh, Howard's not in." Sybil smiled buoyantly. "He's up at the clubhouse, talking with the women."

"Oh, then his ankle's better?"

"No" – her smile wouldn't come off – "he says it's worse. But he's got one of those push things, a walker, and they're all up there discussing doctors and treatments and operations.

"Howard feels real special – he's the only one with both cramps and ankles. He just loves to compare ankles. He couldn't wait to hurry back after lunch, to get a word in first."

I couldn't believe my ears.

"He doesn't worry any more about his advancing age?"

"Heavens, no. He's having a ball! He even told me one of the old ducks now greets him: 'Hello, tiger!' "

. . . and the Screen Doesn't Even Blush

A middle-aged Canadian woman visiting next door complains to me that in Florida she has seen her first video movies "and they made my hair curl. I couldn't believe the goings on and the awful language."

That's understandable if you're over fifty and haven't been keeping up with public entertainment.

Long ago when a magician lifted a rabbit out of a hat, his wide-eyed audience gasped in amazement.

Times have changed.

Today a magician has to cut off his head and walk away with it under his arm before his young audience will stop yawning. Sleight-of-hand artists make automobiles and elephants vanish, and even the Statue of Liberty. What the next bigger stunt will be is a matter of conjecture – unless perhaps it is making the entire world disappear before the Soviets and the Americans do.

Screen fare has undergone an equally revolutionary change. I saw four video movies on a recent weekend; three of them started in bed and spent most of their time there. Hollywood male stars, I learned, don't wear pyjamas any more, possibly because Los Angeles is so warm. And in bed it's even hotter. Hollywood air conditioners are of very poor quality, always going on the blink, because you can hear the couple panting and moaning and thrashing about and never able to find peace.

The only mild movie was *On Golden Pond*, which, however, taught my wife one or two new names to call me when she's angry.

The contrast between screen entertainment in our grandfathers' era and today is strikingly evident in an old yellowed newspaper clipping, pasted in a scrapbook someone gave me. It was from an issue in November 1922, when advertisements offered marble grave monuments for sixty dollars and up, dentists charged "only twenty-five cents per painless extraction," and the newspaper published daily directions on how to tune your tube radio and operate the antenna.

It was the heyday of Walter H. Golding, indefatigable movie promoter from Saint John, New Brunswick. His theatre's big display ad said:

William de Mille's latest Paramount picture at the Imperial – "Nice People" – about what may happen to the modern jazz girl in her pursuit of pleasure-at-any-cost . . . a vital problem of today, presented in a manner both entertaining and artistically perfect.

Wallace Reid plays the role of the young man who is unacquainted with the modern and sophisticated girl.

The ad hints of "a villainess in the movie, a catty young woman" and "a seemingly compromising situation."

But, it concludes,

True Love triumphs in the end, after some trying experiences for the young woman.

Parents, if you have young daughters or sisters, you would do well to take them with you to this movie.

The only difference today is the young daughters decide if the movie is fit to take their parents to.

Give Me Time for My Witty Come-back

When I hold imaginary conversations with friends while I'm out for a walk, I knock them dead with my snappy comebacks. But in real life my friends are very inconsiderate. They don't say the right things to give me a lead-in. They don't let me collect my senses. I never can think of a retort until they have walked away smirking.

The louder they are, the more bewildered I get. For instance, I was telling Frank Fitzdoob in the Pinellas County Volunteer Help Office, where I put in a stint of work occasionally, how I taught my cat to salute with a paw up to her ear.

"You think she's saluting," he snorted. "She's probably scratching her fleas." Several bystanders guffawed, encouraging him to add, "Cats got no intelligence. I could never teach them nothing."

Leaving me groping for words, he strolled chuckling down the hall to the washroom for a smoke.

Then I realized I could have answered, "It's easy. All you need to have is more intelligence than the cat."

I could hardly wait to say it and bring the house down. Pretending to check through a filing cabinet, I watched the door tensely. When he reappeared I called out, "Oh, Frank, speaking about the cat—"

"Who's speaking about the cat?" He grinned around to make sure he had an audience. "I'm not. Say, don't you have anything to do in the office except bring up cats?"

Onlookers snickered. I was helpless to reply, because he had unfairly changed the subject; but I had to keep smiling to show I was enjoying it all immensely.

He swaggered away to the washroom again, laughing at his wittiness. Then it struck me I could answer, "At least, I stay in the office."

I waited grimly for the chance. Glaring at the doorway as I flipped through the files, I was determined to be ready for anything he might say. If he wisecracked, "You'll probably find cat food under *C*," I would pulverize him with, "And you'll probably find Mr. Fitzdoob in the men's washroom." Everyone would roar.

Suddenly I felt a sharp poke in my back. It was a filing drawer, being carried by Frank Fitzdoob, who had evidently come back through another door.

"Better watch out, Tabby," he barked, "or you'll lose one of your nine lives."

I dodged awkwardly, but couldn't think of a thing to say.

"Whatsa matter?" he chortled. "The cat got your tongue?"

And he put on his sun-hat and sauntered out for lunch before I could think to say it certainly didn't have his.

"Anyone Like an Olive?"—Or, How To Enjoy a Jolly Party

An olive, for its size, is a formidable object. It is capable of breaking up a house party. And it can do that even before it is out of the bottle.

The unsuspected powers of the olive usually become apparent at the informal late lunch hour. The hostess, having passed around sandwiches and coffee, calls out from the kitchen as an after-thought: "Anyone like an olive?"

One of the lady guests always tells her yes, but she shouldn't go to all that bother, and she replies it is no bother at all.

A moment later she is sure to poke her head out of the kitchen with: "Who's got good strong hands to turn the top of the olive bottle for me?"

At this the women will protest vigorously that she shouldn't go to so much trouble, and she will say emphatically she is not going to any trouble at all. Meanwhile the men look at each other to see if anyone else is going to get up first.

The host gets up and goes out smiling, with a bantering remark about how wives could never get along without husbands.

Then from the kitchen are heard grunts, followed by muffled exclamations of exasperation, then angry cuss words. A masculine voice seems to be telling somebody that sweet gherkin pickles would have done just as well, or at least the other person might have had enough blasted common sense to have the bottle open before those people barged in.

The guests don't suppose for a minute it is the voice of the host, because he's always such a good-natured fellow. They must be hearing some coarse neighbours through an open window. Nevertheless they feel vaguely uncomfortable.

The host pokes his head out of the kitchen and attempts to grin: "How about one of you fellows trying this trick? My hands are too big to get a grip on the bottle top." He adds weakly, "If it were only a gallon jug, ha, ha . . ."

All three remaining men rise simultaneously, joking and flexing their muscles as they file out to the kitchen, a little embarrassed but not wanting to fail the challenge.

One of them clenches his lips in a tight line, grasps the bottle firmly, and exerts pressure on the cover until his face is apoplectic.

"No good," he gasps. "Hands too warm and slippery. Can't get a decent hold. If I only could keep a hold . . ."

The next man takes a deep breath and a death grip on the bottle, which he holds under this chin, and strains repeatedly to wrench the top around. If he does succeed, his clothes will be showered with olives and juice. Happily, this dawns on him, and he explains, "I don't dare put all my strength into it or I'll get soaked when the top comes off." That lets him out.

The last man, baring his teeth, snatches the bottle from him and snarls furiously at it—"C'mon you, give!"—in the evident hope he will goad it into relaxing its defences and stop trying to hit him back. He doubles up with the bottle hidden somewhere in the pit of his stomach. Anyone outside the kitchen window will have the impression he has taken a violent cramp. Finally he gives up attempting to throttle the bottle, comes out of his cramp, and announces faintly, "I'm afraid to put my full strength to it or I'll smash the glass."

That's one very noticeable similarity between Canadians and Americans at a social party in Florida: no man likes to look like a weakling in front of everyone else.

Everyone is in the kitchen by now, the womenfolk offering earnest advice and criticism, which the men silently endure, though each exhausted husband glares at his wife when she joins in the chorus. Any semblance of cheeriness has long since vanished from the party.

Four broken-spirited men, including the host, eventually shuffle back to the living-room to get away from the scene of their defeat and to explain to each other all over again why it would have been easy if only –

And then the worst happens.

The hostess excitedly appears in the doorway to exclaim, "Clara opened the olives!" Then she darts back to the kitchen, where the women can be heard chattering vivaciously between mouthfuls of olives.

The dismayed men make no move. They just sit there. They never want to hear about olives again. Furthermore, they have all privately decided they don't like Clara, and never did. No one says so, in deference to Clara's husband. But he, too, is wondering why her shrill laughter in the kitchen has such an irritating quality tonight, and is asking himself why he ever married her.

The TV is broadcasting a ball game, and to see the four men absorbed in deep reflection you would feel certain they are following every pitch and batter's swing. The announcer is saying the Red Sox have forty-eight more games on tap.

"She may have held the bottle under the hot water

tap," muses one husband.

The TV voice says the Red Sox rapped in three runs in the second inning.

"Or rapped the cover with a spoon," suggests another husband. "I've seen women do that and you can twist the top right off."

The TV says the Tigers have the experience but the Red Sox have the speed and power.

"It certainly isn't a question of power," adds the host. "It's all in how you turn the cover."

The other husbands readily agree with this and feel somewhat relieved for it. But they begin glumly looking at their watches and saying they had better get their wives out of the kitchen. It is long past time to go home, and tomorrow is a busy day. A man can't do justice to his work if he misses his sleep.

Fortunately, the situation is saved – and the party with it – when the women come into the living-room.

"Wasn't that smart of Clara?" says the hostess. "She just read the directions and do you know what? It turned out to be a bottle you pry the lid off instead of twisting it."

The husbands have a wonderful guffaw over how close they came to crushing the bottle by sheer brute force, with all the muscle they were using. They secretly decide Clara is quite a girl with a lovely lilting laugh.

The party goes on for three hours more. After all, the old gang gets together only once in a dog's age, the husbands point out, so they might as well enjoy themselves. Tomorrow can look after itself.

::

The Meanest Man Living

A ny stranger would think my Florida next-door neighbour Stan was a fine husband, helping around the house, always bringing his wife thoughtful little presents.

Which shows how wrong a chance acquaintance can be.

Stan, who hails from Toronto, is really the meanest man in the world. His wife, Edna, told me so. And he behaves very oddly, too.

My first inkling of the other side of Stan's nature came one day when Edna rushed in from the kitchen and announced eagerly, "There's a man on the phone says I've won a free twenty-nine-dollar ham!"

Stan hardly glanced up from our checkers game.

"Why?" he said. "How did you win it?"

"Oh, some sort of contest, I guess. But I won the ham! All we have to do is both go out to the Vale of Contentment Cemetery, and Mr. Herbert, the representative, will give it to us."

Stan sighed. "I just bet he will." He added, "Tell him you don't want the prize."

Edna looked crestfallen, but after a moment she walked slowly back to the kitchen and I heard her voice: "Thank you just the same, but my husband says he just bought a ham. Goodbye!"

It was the next afternoon, I recall, that Edna rushed into the living-room while we were watching a basketball game on TV.

"I've won again! A bigger prize!"

Still looking at the game, Stan asked, "What is it this time?"

"A free grave!"

"Well," he said, "take it. Jump into it."

Stan, you see, just like me, had been through every kind of high-pressure phone salesmanship for Florida fitness courses, dance lessons, carpet cleaning, water purification, house fumigation – including cemetery salesmen and cremation pushers – since he arrived from Canada for the winter. I'd even known a persistent salesman to phone and ask, out of the blue heavens, "Have you made final arrangements yet?" Once I found to my amazement I was carrying on a conversation with the latest mechanical cremation flack, a telephone recording machine.

But a free grave of my very own – no one had ever offered me that.

"What will I tell Mr. Herbert?" Edna asked. You could see she was eager to own the prize she'd been lucky enough to win.

"There's a catch in it somewhere. Tell him you're not dead yet."

"But, dear! All he wants us to do is go out to the Vale of Contentment and he will show me my grave personally so I can see it is genuine. And then if you sign up for one for yourself, I'll get mine for nothing!"

It was at this point that, for some reason, Stan began to act irrationally.

"That crumb!" he gritted. "He'll drive me into my grave!"

"My grave," she corrected him gently.

"Is he still on the phone?"

"I think so. He's a very obliging gentleman."

Stan leaped out of his chair, ran out, and tore the phone off the wall.

He came back smiling grimly and flopped down in his easy chair to watch the rest of the game.

Smiling – mind you – after losing a ham worth twenty-nine dollars, a grave worth three hundred dollars, and running up a phone repair bill.

"I just feel," he said, "as if I'd won a new lease on life."

Questions that Canadians Ask Most Often

Q: *Where is the best place to change my money into U.S. dollars?*
A: At your own bank before you leave Canada. U.S. banks will usually charge higher rates.

Q: *What is the best season for beach weather in Florida?*
A: November to nearly Christmas; also sometimes into late February, and then again through March and April to mid-May. But a short cold spell will strike either in January or February.

Q: *Is there much difference in temperatures between north and south Florida?*
A: Yes, often. It's a long downward peninsula, and during the winter the Fahrenheit readings may be twenty degrees chillier around Pensacola in the north than at Key West on the southern tip.

Q: *Has metric made any noticeable impact on Florida?*
A: No. Most highway speed signs showing metric as well

as miles per hour have disappeared. Liquors and wines are sold in metric measurement, but supermarket and department store goods are weighed in pounds and ounces, and measured in yards. Gas stations yielded to public pressure and changed pumps back from litres to gallons.

The U.S., in a sense, clings to British traditions more steadfastly than Canada does. Big residential developments are called "Windsor Downs," "Canterbury Heights," and a thousand other majestic names. A vehement fight is being waged on the Atlantic side to make English the official language of Florida – which provokes charges of "racism" from the well-entrenched Hispanic population.

Miami thought the huge influx of Cubans, Colombians, Nicaraguans, Venezuelans, and others would be absorbed into the great American melting pot. It wasn't. You can be born, get an education, watch TV, read daily papers, live, and die entirely in Spanish. Dade County's Hispanic population will climb in this decade to over a million; for it already far outnumbers English-speaking whites and blacks together.

If I made a guess, I'd say the U.S. – including the Mexican-Americans – will ultimately become a bilingual nation, English- and Spanish-speaking, and the Hispanics will be in the majority.

Q: *How safe for tourists is the gun-toting Atlantic coast?*
A: Reasonably safe – if you walk in a park at night with a Great Dane on a leash. Everyone is trying to find a way to cope with the epidemic of police and court corruption, cocaine-related stabbings, gangland revenge slayings, race riots, pedestrian muggings, and burglaries. Mayor Spero Canton of Miami Shores thinks he has the best idea. He'd erect huge concrete barricades in front of most of his city's streets to keep the criminals out – a throwback to moats and drawbridges, to Hadrian's Wall and the Great Wall of China.

Paradoxically, as mobsters and police officers keep falling to the hail fire from smugglers' guns, the state of Florida is handing out permits for carrying concealed weapons at the rate of four thousand a month. And some legal authorities point out that due to an unfortunate lack of precise wording in the law, sub-machine-guns, too, can be carried as "concealed weapons." Meanwhile, children of gun owners occasionally carry loaded revolvers to school to impress all their classmates – and sometimes merely to shoot specific bullies or teachers.

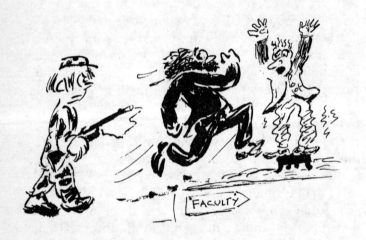

Q: *How are retail prices?*
A: Gasoline is still much cheaper than in Canada – about half to two-thirds of our prices, as low as ninety-nine cents a U.S. gallon. Wines, liquor, and beer are also bargains. A three-litre jug of Carlo Rossi California wine is $4.99. However, clothing in the two countries is closing the price gap, counting the Florida 6-per-cent tax; but Canadians find the variety is still far wider and sprightlier in the south. New car prices are holding the line or even dropping, which reflects the intense competition of overstocks. Supermarket prices have risen, but not by more than twenty or thirty cents extra for a package of cereal.

Q: *Are homes scarce to buy or rent on the Suncoast?*
A: No. They're plentiful – a reaction perhaps to the vast hotel building boom near Tampa's popular Busch Gardens, Sea World and its new penguin colony, Disney World, with its new movie-making studios and nightly sky laser show, and Spaceport U.S.A. at Cape Canaveral. Also, when interest rates go up, mortgages are hard for young couples to get. Few can lay down the cash price.

Q: *Is it useful to have Canadian Automobile Association membership?*
A: Yes, very. Their offices will compile detailed travel Triptiks for you, make your hotel and motel reservations, sell you American Express traveller's cheques without charge, among other things.

When our car battery conked out after the inside lights were left on all night, I phoned the Seminole AAA. They said they'd send help. I asked, "What day, so I can arrange to be here?" The reply: "Within twenty minutes." The truck was waiting for me in ten. On a really cold January day, I was told, the local AAA may be called in to do 1,500 free booster jobs.

Q: *If you were planning to live permanently in Florida, where would you locate?*
A: Probably in a more southerly area, where traffic would be less – for the moment.

Today, when an accident occurs on one of the three bridges and causeways leading across Tampa Bay from St. Petersburg to the Tampa airport, you may be blocked for as long as four hours – and you can say goodbye to your airliner leaving Tampa airport in an hour. They're even talking of founding a complete new city next door in Pasco County, ultimately adding 98,000 car trips a day to the congested roads.

But you become attached to your own community. I rent a villa in a quiet senior complex where, if you haven't got a pace-maker or at least a walker, you're not in the social club. A dual pace-maker is a real status symbol, entitling you to gloat over ordinary residents.

It's a very central place. If I wish, I can drive a few miles and take a trip in a balloon, soar in a sailplane, swim with the dolphins or manatees, ride an elephant, go deep-sea fishing, take a Caribbean cruise, see Broadway shows or the Ringling Bros. Barnum and Bailey Circus.

Q: *Are there plenty of good inexpensive restaurants for average tourists?*
A: Are there ever! One or two new ones open on the Gulf of Mexico Suncoast every day (and one or two close). Oddly, some elite dining spots are exasperatingly slow because the waiter puts on a show of flashing carving knives over his head at other tables as he serves from his trolley. By the time he starts his flashing act at your table, your costly dinner is stone-cold – and you may or may not have the courage to send it back.

Or the tiny printing at the bottom of the menu will say 15 per cent gratuity is added to your bill, but in the dim candlelight you don't notice and leave another 15 per cent.

A sure guarantee of popularity, it seems, is to give the place a bizarre name. Crabby Bill's at Indian Rocks Beach did so well it expanded into several nearby buildings. As a lark, yuppies sit on long wooden benches and pound open their shellfish by banging mallets, while dodging spray from other diners' mallets in the continuous din.

A nearby newer restaurant is Fast Eddie's, one of a chain famous in the west for its slogan of "Warm Beer and Lousy Food." This is sheer magnetism for the young crowd. Naturally, no one can ever complain about anything even if he wants to – the waiters need only point to the motto.

I hadn't heard about the fast-growing Ya-Ya sit-down-or-take-out eateries which specialize in delicious flame-broiled chicken. So when we took friends of ours, an old-time New Brunswick newspaper co-worker and his wife, back to their St. Petersburg home after lunch uptown, he asked me earnestly:

"Would you like to go to the Ya-Ya?"

"No, thanks," I said, in surprise. "I think I'll be all right till I get home."

It's North America in Miniature

Florida, as advance pollsters point out during presidential elections, isn't really a Southern state. It's a microcosm of all states and provinces, and therefore a political barometer.

The first question you ask on making a new acquaintance is, "Where was your original home?" To be a native-born Floridian is a badge of distinction.

A thousand newcomers a day arrive in Florida to live; and even if a few hundred a day die of old age or otherwise leave to return home, it's still a big boost to the population.

A fez-hatted Shriner at a Clearwater luncheon confided to me, "Every new family adds to the traffic jams, air pollution, loss of natural environment. So every newcomer wants to shut the gate on any more people moving in."

Life-styles are widely varied. There are old settled communities, seasonal concentrations of hundreds of trailer homes, smaller parks of homey mom-and-pop couples in mobile homes (often name-plated "Archie Loves Maybelle" or "The Happy Nest of Gerry and Liz Bird"), well-run condominium complexes for seniors, imposing private homes, and at the Palm Beach island resort in the south, luxurious estates which sometimes have more than a hundred rooms and are worth tens of millions.

But the ultra-self-indulgent life of much satirized Palm Beach – called by the German magazine *Der Stern* "The Paradise of the Living Dead" – palls on many of the wealthy widows who exist there. Some look as if they've already spent their ten bonus years on periodic face-lifts. Accompanied by their beautifully groomed Hispanic-looking young men – hired personal escorts – they attend three formal balls a week for good causes each winter. The monotony of it all is reflected in the jaded laugh of one lavishly bejewelled widow who asked a friend, "Who are we dancing for tonight?"

Banks, Lawyers, Doctors, Hospitals, Churches, and Graves

The difference between life in Florida and in Canada begins to vanish from your consciousness once you get accustomed to seeing an apparent nineteen-year-old blonde with a wild frazzled hair-do strolling along in shiny skin-tight leotards patterned in a huge medieval-style diamond design – and, when she turns around, discovering she's a wrinkled seventy-nine-year-old grandmother.

On the beach they're all teenagers – from a distance.

And we quickly get used to distinctive words, phrases, and inflections. "Have a nice day" has been imported into Canada, but not yet "It's a pretty day" or "*in*quiry" (they pronounce it "*en*querry"), "in*flu*ence" or "de*tails*." We say Boy *Scout*, they say *Boy* Scout and *peanut* butter, *oat*meal, *bean* soup. We can't hear ourselves uttering, "eh?" or a harsh Scottish "about" as Americans claim, any more than they can hear the strident nasal voices of many U.S. women TV commentators.

There was a time I imagined that all local accents in Britain would be ironed out by the invasion of U.S. radio, movies, and TV. Now all I hear in high-class American-made movies and TV plays and in TV commercials are English voices – that is, when they aren't Canadian voices.

It's just a question of who's taking over whom.

A similar question underlies the great modern invasion of Canadian investment capital in the United States. Toronto and Montreal financiers have poured billions into acquiring U.S. department-store chains, real estate, distilleries, breweries, banks, theatres, even orange juice.

It's won new respect in the U.S. for the northern snowbirds, formerly thought of as a dullish people who amused themselves mostly by sending down wintry weather blasts to give their good neighbours to the south a freezing jolt.

Canadians, in turn, are still baffled by the U.S. temperament. They look on in wonderment at the highly volatile emotionalism of this land where a man can be a national hero one day and something less the next day, where unfurling the Stars and Stripes to the accompaniment of "God Bless America" is a national obsession. "It's as though they just won their freedom last year and are worried about losing it," a tourist from Winnipeg mused. But at the same time he admitted he himself knew only the first line of "O Canada."

If Canadians have been hesitant about closer relations with the United States, it's because they're traditionally wary of being trapped in any cross-the-border agreement from which they can't escape – trapped by loud-voiced complaints from huge U.S. industries or dominated by U.S. government agencies, like the Pentagon, and losing their cultural independence in the bargain.

Because many Florida retirees are rich as well as decrepit, uptown street corners have been monopolized by banks as well as the ubiquitous gas stations. Churches and cemeteries take a back pew, but they're both thronged nevertheless. Mortgage lenders, real estate dealers, re-

ducing salons, dentists, doctors, and hospitals are everywhere. The countless osteopaths (DOs) run their own large
Suncoast Hospital. And ever keenly alert are dozens of
law firms proclaiming their speed in getting New Year's
Eve drunken-driving arrests and accident claims settled
for a cut of the cash – "first consultation free."

But the majority of Canadians admire and like our
American cousins, despite their overbearing reputation
and the acquisitive win-at-any-cost tactics that often spur
them on. As a college basketball coach announced: "We're
not in it to play the game – we're in it to win." And a
new National League football club owner said: "We play
to win. There's no substitute for that."

The Americans, reciprocating the good will, envy Canada's "socialized medicine" and the fact that our national
revenue department doesn't grab a share of everyone's
winnings on lotteries and game shows. And U.S tourists
write hundreds of letters to Canadian newspapers every
year expressing their appreciation for the helpfulness they
encountered on Canadian vacation tours.

Watching a Play Isn't Easy with a Strange Girl in Your Lap

On our way to Florida we stopped in New York, and decided to splurge on a Broadway show. It cost us a hundred dollars for two seats, which proved to be tight knee-squeezers in the first balcony, right under the amplified voice of the "stage director"; the script called for him to keep shouting insults at the female star, who was supposed to be an old flame of his. This was disconcerting enough from the start.

Beside me sat my wife, and beyond her a half-dozen Japanese teenagers with their ageing mentor. They were having a ball in New York, these giggling girls, all so cute as they showed each other their souvenir brochures.

Then, halfway through the play, one girl got up to go out, probably to check on their car.

She squeezed by my wife somehow, but as I was securely wedged in, I couldn't make room for her.

Finally, she turned her back to me, flung one leg over

my knees – and then tried to get past by flinging the other leg over, too.

It didn't work.

She fell into my lap.

I struggled to haul her up, and she grabbed the seat arms – all to no avail.

Time after time she almost made it, then tumbled back.

Here I was, in a Broadway theatre with a comely girl sitting in my lap. What a compromising picture for any unscrupulous photographer to take and blackmail me with! But fortunately my wife was right there beside me, shoving mightily and urging, "Do something! Do something!"

Do what?

In a desperate last effort – I hated to do it, because people were watching – I squeezed my hands down under her to hoist up my visitor bodily; and you know an odd thing? She looked fairly chubby but she must have weighed a ton. Her underside seemed to be made of cast iron. I might as well have tried to lift the *Queen Mary*.

At last the couple in the end seats got out into the aisle to pull too. And due to the efforts of five people – my wife, the girl, myself, and the two benefactors – the victim was lifted to freedom.

What still puzzles me, however, is that lovely Japanese girl. She must have had difficulties in locating their car, because she never came back.

... so 'Bye for Now, Florida

Florida newspapers are full of "eat as much as you want" restaurant ads, which encourage you to gorge yourself, and of large ads promoting clinics to take off weight.

In a big mall parking lot filled with hundreds of automobiles, you'll see a car full of fat ladies circling around and around for five minutes to find a spot nearer the front door so they won't have to walk so far. Then they squeeze out of the car, amble into the mall, and head for their weight reduction salon to start jogging.

The most welcome visitor in Florida residential complexes isn't Santa, but the daily postal carrier.

Householders know the sound of the mail driver's car engine, and come in a rush.

The scene is usually the same: The ageing grandparent stumbling back from the community mailboxes with an armload of big envelopes, muttering, "Just junk, junk, and more junk."

They'll tell you their grandchildren never write, nor

even thank them for presents. If the kids want a special favour, like an invitation to bring some classmates down for the Easter break, they'll phone – collect.

The selling strategy of booths in a giant St. Petersburg flea market is intriguing.

"Shoes and Boots up to Size 17. Also Sole Cushions," proclaims a sign. It's eleven A.M. and few shoppers have stopped. Comments the dealer, "Wait till mid-afternoon – that's when their feet start killing them from all the walking."

Another sign: "Used False Teeth – Fit Guaranteed." And folks actually buy them – despite dentists' angry warnings that you can't get fitted over the counter: "There's as much difference between people's gums as between people's fingerprints."

Why Floridians admire Canada's medicare:

The wisp of a girl helping clean our apartment phoned home to ask her mother-in-law whether the baby was all right.

"I suppose you'll have six kids by the time we come back next winter," I said jokingly.

"No," she replied. "We have to save for a year or two. We're just a young couple with no insurance, and it cost us $2,500 to have the baby here in St. Petersburg." She added cheerfully, "But we were lucky – we'd have had to pay $3,000 in Tampa."

The speed of Florida developers can be breathtaking.

Go to a supermarket to shop, and you return to find the avenue newly bordered with towering ornamental palm trees.

Take a two-week sea cruise – and you find luxurious $250,000 homes have suddenly mushroomed all over a former orange grove next door, complete with a large horseshoe-shaped lake, water fountains, and real live white egrets.

But Florida can't operate its Crystal River nuclear plant without continual breakdowns. On my arrival one November I found it had been "down" longer than in operation that year. And the giant new Sunshine Skyway bridge construction project was plagued by problems for years. Finally, discovering the bridge floor was too high, they pulled down the ends with cables to fit the pavement.

Perhaps it will take feminine inventiveness to make life more efficient in Florida – like a middle-aged woman my daughter-in-law met in a ladies' rest room at Disney World. Everyone was freezing that frosty January day – everyone but the middle-aged woman.

"See?" she explained to the others. "I've got a wool sweater on upside down, with my legs down through the arms and the front buttoned up over my stomach. I'm warm as toast!"

Her ingenuity brought shrieks of admiration, and also predictions that in the next cold spell a lot of husbands' sweaters would disappear.

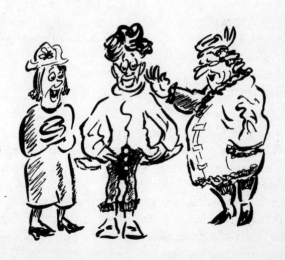

And lastly – perhaps fittingly, on a note of finality:

Florida funeral homes and last resting places are livelier than ever.

A friend who drove up the Gulf of Mexico coast the other evening reported passing a brightly illuminated highway-side cemetery with a message spelled out in electric lights:

"Now 60,000 Members."

It neglected to say whether they were signed-up future occupants or permanent residents already enjoying the good afterlife there.